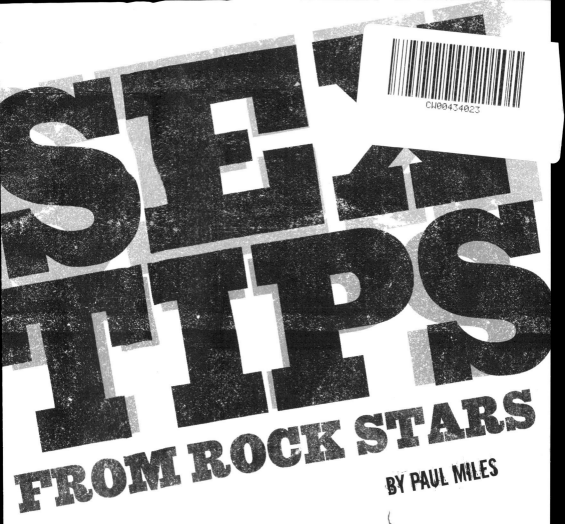

SEX TIPS

FROM ROCK STARS

BY PAUL MILES

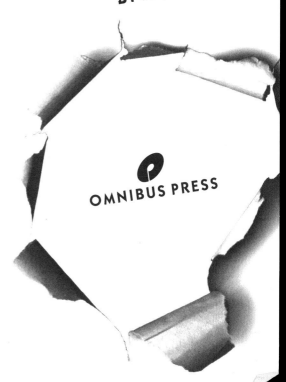

OMNIBUS PRESS

Cover and book designed by Fresh Lemon

ISBN: 978.1 .84938.404.9
Order No: OP 53427

Exclusive Distributors
Music Sales Limited,
14/15 Berners Street,
London, W1T 3LJ.

Music Sales Corporation,
257 Park Avenue South,
New York, NY 10010, USA.

Macmillan Distribution Services,
56 Parkwest Drive
Derrimut, Vic 3030,
Australia.

Printed by: Gutenberg Press Ltd, Malta.

A catalogue record for this book is available from the British Library.

Visit Omnibus Press on the web at www.omnibuspress.com

For more information on *Sex Tips From Rock Stars,*
please visit www.SexTipsFromRockStars.com.

CONTENTS

WHY DO ROCK STARS PULL THE HOTTIES?

"THE MOST OUTRAGEOUS WAS PROBABLY WHEN A CHICK JUMPED UP ONSTAGE AND BLEW ME WHILE WE WERE PLAYING"

All over the modern world, there are millions of people either playing in bands or as solo artists. Most are just dabbling in it; some are putting their all into trying to 'make it'. But the odds of success are incredibly low (just as AC/DC dutifully educated us in the lyrics to 'It's a Long Way to the Top'.)

Music is a tough industry and it seems to be getting even tougher to earn a decent living as a rock'n'roll musician. Those that fail in the pursuit typically look for more secure employment and dabble again on the side, often hoping they'll get another shot. For those that do make it and get to play in a rock band that tours the world, fame awaits.

And with this fame comes power – and what an aphrodisiac power is! When a rock star takes the stage and strikes an opening guitar chord, or thumps a familiar drum beat, or wails through the microphone "Hello [insert city name here]", the cheers and screams from thousands of concert-goers reverberate around the venue. A performing rock star has the power to make each person in their crowd smile and be happy, make them lose themselves in the moment, and make them feel fantastic – even euphoric.

This creates instantaneous high-level interest within many of the opposite sex and they want to get closer. Many go weak at the knees, buckling to the power of the rock star under the spotlight. It's a big turn-on, subconsciously or not.

Thus the logic extends that if a) you're able to meet the rock star, b) there's a mutual attraction, c) you get it on with them, and d) you keep the relationship going, then your life is going to be pretty damn cool and full of satisfaction. Knowing that countless other people also desire this from the rock star brings out the competitive juices and increases the magnetism.

The allure of their fame can also turn rational, well-balanced humans into crazed psychos on heat. It also attracts other undesirables along the way. So it's no wonder the rock star has 'people' that act as a filter designed to only let the most all-round attractive prospects through to the rock star's domain. But this only amplifies the challenge for some. (You'll get to learn plenty of tips for this shortly.)

Knowing that rock stars only allow the best-of-the-best into their world – people who are primed to please – means they're revered as powerful stars that experience amazing sexual situations that others can only dream about.

But what is their world *really* like? Well, that's the question this book answers: it gives *you* backstage access into the real lives of rock stars and what they actually see, try, experience and recommend when it comes to every aspect of sex. It's part eroticism, part rock biography, part comedy and part self-help.

But be warned: chances are you'll find yourself in a future sexual situation and at least one of the tips from this book will likely come to mind! (I hope it's a good one.)

So slap that VIP pass on and follow me as I host your entertaining Q&A session with twenty-three international rock stars that are ready to share their ideas and thoughts on all of their sexual instincts, urges and experiences with you.

THE ROCK STARS

> "I FUCKING HATE CONDOMS. THEY'RE A NECESSARY EVIL, BUT CONDOMS ARE FOR GUYS WITH SHORT HAIR!"

1. **Acey Slade (Murderdolls/Dope)**

2. Adde (Hardcore Superstar)

3. **Allison Robertson (The Donnas)**

4. Andrew W.K.

5. **Blasko (Ozzy Osbourne/Rob Zombie)**

6. Brent Muscat (Faster Pussycat)

7. **Bruce Kulick (Kiss/Grand Funk Railroad)**

8. Chip Z'Nuff (Enuff Z'Nuff)

9. **Courtney Taylor-Taylor (The Dandy Warhols)**

10. Danko Jones

11. **Doug Robb (Hoobastank)**

12. Evan Seinfeld (Biohazard)

13. **Ginger (The Wildhearts)**

14. Handsome Dick Manitoba (The Dictators/MC5)

15. **James Kottak (Scorpions/Kingdom Come)**

16. Jesse Hughes (Eagles of Death Metal)

17. **Jimmy Ashhurst (Buckcherry)**

18. Joel O'Keeffe (Airbourne)

19. **Lemmy (Motörhead)**

20. Nicke Borg (Backyard Babies)

21. **Rob Patterson (Korn/Otep)**

22. Toby Rand (Juke Kartel)

23. **Vazquez (Damone)**

ACEY SLADE (b 1974)

Acey Slade is a multi-talented rock star hailing from Pennsylvania, USA. After fronting the Vampire Love Dolls, he joined Dope in 1999 as their bass player and toured America several times supporting their major label debut, *Felons & Revolutionaries,* for Epic Records. Acey moved to guitar for the band's follow-up album, *Life,* which landed in the Billboard 200 chart, before leaving Dope in the middle of 2002 to be a guitarist in the Murderdolls. The band released their album *Beyond The Valley Of The Murderdolls* and took their unique combination of horror punk and glam metal on tour through the US, Japan, Europe and Australia. While collaborating with fellow Murderdolls guitarist Joey Jordison (better known as the drummer in Slipknot) on a track celebrating Roadrunner Records' 25-year anniversary, Acey was also busy fronting his own band, Trashlight Vision. Performing lead vocals and guitar on two EPs and the album *Alibis And Ammunition,* Acey again toured across the US, Europe and Japan before disbanding Trashlight Vision in 2007. He has since been in the studio producing Scottish acoustic punk band Billy Liar, and working on new music for his next band, Acey Slade & The Dark Party. After releasing two EPs, the band released their self-titled, full-length album early in 2010.

ADDE (b 1976)

Magnus 'Adde' Andreasson is the founding drummer for Hardcore Superstar, a rock/metal band from Gothenburg, Sweden. Formed in 1997, the band has had several number one hit singles and earned multiple Grammy nominations in their homeland. They have been on all major national music TV and radio shows in Sweden and enjoyed successful tours of Europe, North America, Japan and Australia. Adde spent an eye-opening period of his life studying at the Musicians Institute in Los Angeles. With their fused brand of sleaze rock and thrash metal, Hardcore Superstar won the Swedish Metal Award for Best Hard Rock Album of the Year in 2007 for *Dreamin' in a Casket.* Their next album, *Beg For It,* was released mid-2009 after first single, the title track, went gold in Sweden and debuted at number five on the national charts. Adde continues to tour with Hardcore Superstar to this day, enjoying the resurgence in the band's career.

ALLISON ROBERTSON (b 1979)

Allison Robertson plays guitar in the Californian all-female hard rock band The Donnas. Starting to play guitar at 12, she soon formed a band with her best school friends, touring Japan for the first time during their senior year of high school. After a string of singles, The Donnas released four full-length albums on Lookout Records between 1997 and 2001 before earning major label commercial success with Atlantic Records. Their next album, *Spend The Night,* hit number 62 on the *Billboard* charts and features their most successful single, 'Take It Off', which peaked at number 19 on *Billboard*'s Modern Rock chart. After touring on the main stage of the Lollapalooza festival in 2003, their sixth album, *Gold Medal,* was released the following year. The single 'Fall Behind Me' was featured in TV commercials and performed live in the TV series *Charmed.* Their songs also feature on many movie soundtracks and video games, including *Guitar Hero* and *Rock Band.* The Donnas released their next album, *Bitchin',* on their own Purple Feather Records in 2007, when it spent a month on *Billboard*'s charts as they toured as far as Australia. While The Donnas prepared their next release, entitled *Greatest Hits, Volume 16,* Allison teamed up with former Hole and Nashville Pussy members in a new all-female covers band named Chelsea Girls. Attracting media attention with their first three sold-out shows at The Roxy in Los Angeles, they secured a monthly residency at the legendary venue. The Donnas then joined Blondie and Pat Benatar on a summer 2009 tour across the US.

ANDREW W.K. (b 1979)

Multi-talented American rock musician Andrew Wilkes-Krier first came to prominence with his self-produced major label solo debut, *I Get Wet,* in 2001, which hit number one on *Billboard*'s Heatseekers chart. The controversial cover art features a photo of Andrew with blood streaming from his nose to his throat. With the track 'Party Hard' getting lots of radio airplay, Andrew toured on Ozzfest. Tracks from the album made their way into several video games, plus movie and TV soundtracks. His follow-up, *The Wolf,* also reached the *Billboard* 200 and featured Andrew playing all the instruments; the song 'Long Live The Party' was a minor hit in Japan. Universal Music then released his J-Pop album, *The Japan Covers,* instigated by 20,000 plus sales of his chart-topping ringtones in Japan. A solo piano album called *55 Cadillac* was released in 2009 on his own record label, Skyscraper Music Maker. Outside his solo music, Andrew has performed as a self-help, new age motivational speaker; produces music for other artists (everything from reggae to an avant-garde ensemble); and has played various instruments on other artists' recordings. As *Time* magazine was calling him 'truly cute' in 2008, Andrew and three partners opened the multi-level nightclub and live concert hall Santos Party House in Manhattan, New York City. Andrew has also had his own shows on MTV, called *Crashing With Andrew W.K.* and *Your Friend, Andrew W.K.* He partnered with the Cartoon Network in 2009 to host and create music for a new live action TV show called *Destroy Build Destroy.*

BLASKO (b 1969)

Rob 'Blasko' Nicholson is an American hard rock bassist best known for his work with Rob Zombie and Ozzy Osbourne. Blasko began his career playing bass for the speed/thrash metal band Cryptic Slaughter, before moving on to Prong and Danzig. He left Danzig to tour with Rob Zombie and has played on all of the latter's platinum-selling solo albums to date, which have sold more than 15 million copies worldwide. In 2003, Blasko replaced Robert Trujillo as

Ozzy Osbourne's bassist, becoming a full-time member with Ozzy's ninth studio album, *Black Rain,* which debuted at number three on the *Billboard* charts (Ozzy's highest debut to date). The album's first single, 'I Don't Wanna Stop', reached number one on *Billboard*'s Hot Mainstream Rock chart in 2007 (another first for Ozzy) and was nominated for a 2008 Grammy Award for Best Hard Rock Performance. Today, Blasko continues to tour the world with Ozzy and also runs his own music management and consultancy business, Mercenary Management, where he manages the band In This Moment among others.

BRENT MUSCAT (b 1967)

Brent is a founding member of Hollywood hard rock band Faster Pussycat. Elektra Records signed the band and released their self-titled debut album in 1987 when the androgynous-looking guitarist was just 20 years old. The band contributed a now-revered live performance in the classic Sunset Strip rock film *The Decline Of Western Civilization Part II The Metal Years* before touring around North America with Alice Cooper, David Lee Roth and Motörhead. The band's follow-up album, *Wake Me When It's Over*, is their most successful to date, selling over half-a-million copies in the US and being certified gold status. With the hit single 'House Of Pain' being spun on many radio stations, Faster Pussycat toured with Kiss and Mötley Crüe before recording a cover of 'You're So Vain' to help celebrate Elektra's 40th Anniversary. Brent continued to play with Faster Pussycat until 2005, when a diagnosis of oral cancer triggered his unceremonious departure from the band. Now in remission, Brent enjoys rocking Las Vegas casino stages with his own band, Sin City Sinners, and an all-star rock'n'roll cast of players.

BRUCE KULICK (b 1953)

Bruce is an American guitarist who began his international rock career on Meat Loaf's *Bat Out Of Hell* world tour during 1977-78, before playing on Billy Squier and Michael Bolton albums in the early Eighties. Bruce was then the lead guitarist for hard rock band Kiss from 1984 until 1996, for which he is best known. After joining Kiss for the *Animalize* tour, their next three albums in the Eighties (*Asylum*, *Crazy Nights* and *Smashes, Thrashes & Hits*) were all certified platinum. The band consistently toured all over the globe and as the Nineties rolled around, Kiss' next albums (*Hot In The Shade*, *Revenge* and *Kiss Unplugged*) all went gold. When the original Kiss members reunited in 1996, Bruce left to form Union with former Mötley Crüe frontman John Corabi. Union released three albums and a live DVD and toured through the US, Europe, Australia and Central America. Since 2001, Bruce has been the lead guitarist in Grand Funk Railroad, the rock band that was highly popular in the Seventies and best-known for their number one hit 'We're An American Band'. Bruce has also released three solo albums: *Audio Dog* in 2001, *Transformer* in 2003, and *BK3* in 2010.

CHIP Z'NUFF

Chip Z'Nuff is the bassist and driving force behind the much-gifted power pop band Enuff Z'Nuff. After forming in Chicago in 1984, they released their self-titled debut album on an Atlantic Records subsidiary five years later. The album's two minor, psychedelic-tinged, hit singles, 'New Thing' and 'Fly High Michelle', received steady radio airplay and rotations on MTV, while Chip's brief intimate liaison with Madonna was fodder for popular shock-jock and long-time fan Howard Stern. Toning down their colourful image, Enuff Z'Nuff released a fan-favourite album, *Strength,* in 1991 to strong reviews and performed live on *The Late Show With David Letterman.* With musical climate changes and subsequent disappointing sales, Enuff Z'Nuff fell out with their label but were quickly signed by Arista Records, producing one album in 1993 as personnel problems unsettled the band. Despite setbacks including band members dying from cancer and a drug overdose, Enuff Z'Nuff has built a solid international fan base – particularly in Japan – through consistent touring and independent album releases. As work continues on Enuff Z'Nuff's 15th album, Chip is also a judge of the world's best marijuana in the Cannabis Cup for *High Times* magazine. He also has his own label, Stoney Records, and is performing and recording with the band Adler's Appetite featuring former Guns N' Roses drummer Steven Adler.

COURTNEY TAYLOR-TAYLOR (b 1967)

Courtney Taylor-Taylor is the lead singer, guitarist and principal songwriter for the American alternative rock band The Dandy Warhols. Their first album, *Dandys Rule, OK?,* was released in 1995 and caught the ears of major label Capitol Records, which signed them. Their next release came two years later, when the band was selling out concerts across Europe and Australia. The new millennium brought a new album, *Thirteen Tales From Urban Bohemia*, which reached platinum status in Australia, the UK and other European countries. The song 'Bohemian Like You' was used extensively by Vodafone in a successful TV campaign that propelled the single to number five on the UK charts. The band's music has been used in many advertising campaigns, TV series and movies ever since. The Dandy Warhols' other big single is 'We Used To Be Friends' (featuring Nick Rhodes from Duran Duran on synthesizer) from their *Welcome To The Monkey House* album of 2003. The band continues to write and record albums at 'The Odditorium' – their large multi-purpose studio in hometown Portland, Oregon.

DANKO JONES

Danko Jones is the charismatic singer and guitarist in the hard rock band of the same name. Formed in Toronto in 1996, the three-piece gigged consistently while Danko also worked in a sex shop. Their self-produced second EP, *My Love Is Bold,* was nominated for Best Alternative Album in Canada's 2000 Juno

Awards. Bad Taste Records in Sweden signed them the following year and they completed three tours of Europe before 2002, when their first full-length album, *Born A Lion,* was released. The band again completed several European tours and two Canadian tours, including a hometown opening slot with The Rolling Stones. The next Danko Jones album, *We Sweat Blood*, received a 2003 Juno nomination for Best Rock Album. The band toured for three years throughout Europe, Japan, Australia, North America and South Africa while putting together their next album, *Sleep Is The Enemy*. During this time, Danko also released his first spoken-word album, *The Magical World Of Rock,* and completed two spoken-word tours to support it. The hard-working band toured Canadian arenas with Nickelback in 2006 before hitting America and European festivals, releasing a *Live In Stockholm* DVD in the process. They again toured heavily behind 2008's *Never Too Loud* album and their 2009 *B-sides* collection. Danko writes four separate bi-monthly columns for European rock magazines and continues to host his own radio show, *The Magical World of Rock*, broadcast from Sweden and syndicated to stations in Europe and Canada.

DOUG ROBB (b 1975)

Born to a Japanese mother and a Scottish father, Douglas Robb is the lead singer of the Southern Californian alternative rock band Hoobastank, who have sold more than five million albums worldwide to date since forming in 1994. Signing to Island Records in 2000 after a couple of self-produced discs, the band soon released a self-titled album for the label containing their breakthrough hit, 'Crawling In The Dark'. Propelled by chart success, the album went platinum and the band toured across America, Europe and Asia, before they were invited to play in the Rock and Roll Hall of Fame. The title track of their next album, *The Reason,* became a massive hit worldwide in 2004, reaching number two on the *Billboard* Hot 100 and spending 21 weeks at the top of Canada's singles chart – a new record for most weeks at number one. The song was played during the final episode of the TV series *Friends*, while the album reached number three on the *Billboard* 200 chart, was certified multi-platinum and received three Grammy nominations. The band has continued to tour the world and release new studio albums since – *Every Man For Himself* in 2006 has been certified gold, and *For(N)ever* in 2009 – both of which have landed in the *Billboard* 200 album chart.

EVAN SEINFELD (b 1967)

Formed in Brooklyn during 1987 by bassist and vocalist Evan Seinfeld, Biohazard are acknowledged as one of the earliest bands to fuse hardcore punk and heavy metal with elements of hip hop music. The band's 1992 album, *Urban Discipline,* sold more than a million copies worldwide, propelled by the video for the song 'Punishment', which became the most-played video in the history of MTV's *Headbanger's Ball*. Their next album also sold in excess of one million copies and the band toured the world once again. Evan began an acting career in 1998, playing Jaz Hoyt on HBO's award-winning series *Oz*. Porn star Tera Patrick saw one of his nude scenes on *Oz* and the two soon struck up a relationship before marrying in 2004. In 2006, Evan participated in the VH-1 reality television series *Supergroup* that also starred Ted Nugent, Scott Ian, Sebastian Bach and Jason Bonham as a band named Damnocracy. Evan still plays concerts with Biohazard, as well as with his new band, The Spyderz. Using the alias Spyder Jones, Evan has starred in and directed many adult movies. His rockstarpimp.com website is the world's only celebrity rock star porn site. Note: Some months after Evan's interview for this book, he and Tera announced their separation.

GINGER (b 1964)

The Wildhearts are a rock band formed in late 1989 in Newcastle-upon-Tyne, England, following Ginger's sacking from The Quireboys. Throughout their turbulent and unpredictable history, The Wildhearts have remained at the forefront of the British rock scene. The only constant member has been the band's founder Ginger, who is the group's singer, guitarist and predominant songwriter. Despite several Top 20 singles and one Top 10 album in England, The Wildhearts have missed out on major commercial success, owing in part to difficulties with record companies and many internal problems, often relating to recreational drugs and depression. Ginger has also embarked upon a variety of solo and side projects over the years. The Wildhearts' energetic live performances in recent times (including their show-stealing performance at 2008's Download Festival) have seen the band's popularity hit new heights as they tour worldwide and cement their reputation and legacy as one of the best rock bands the UK has ever produced. 2009 saw the release of their ninth studio album, *¡Chutzpah!,* before the band embarked on yet another tour.

HANDSOME DICK MANITOBA (b 1954)

In 1975, Richard 'Handsome Dick' Manitoba (aka The Handsomest Man in Rock'n'Roll) became the singer for The Dictators, the legendary New York City proto-punk band. The band's loud, hard, fast sound combined with junk culture lyrics created a rock'n'roll archetype that has inspired and influenced countless other bands, including The Ramones. Many considered The Dictators to be the first punk band from the New York scene to have an album released on a major label. The Handsome One opened his world-famous NYC rock bar, named Manitoba's, early in '99, and it remains an East Village institution. Since early 2005, Manitoba has been lead singer for The MC5, the iconic Detroit pre-punk rock'n'roll band most famous for their classic song 'Kick Out The Jams'. In 2006, The Dictators played the last-ever Friday and Saturday nights at the legendary punk rock venue CBGB's. Dick is also a radio personality, currently hosting *The Handsome Dick Manitoba Radio Program* on Little Steven Van Zandt's Underground Garage channel on Sirius XM Radio.

JAMES KOTTAK (b 1962)

James Kottak is an American drummer who first came to prominence in the hard rock band Kingdom Come. Their self-titled debut album, released in 1988, sounded remarkably like early Led Zeppelin and success of the first single, 'Get It On', helped the album go platinum in many countries, including Germany, Canada and the US. They toured on the Monsters of Rock festival, and supported Scorpions on two tours. James left Kingdom Come soon after their second album, before playing drums on albums by MSG and Warrant. He also formed his own punk band, Krunk, alongside wife Athena (sister of Mötley Crüe's Tommy Lee) on drums. With James on lead vocals and guitar, they were awarded Best Punk Band in Los Angeles in 1997 and they continue playing today under the name Kottak. Since 1996 James has been the drummer for Scorpions, the German heavy metal/hard rock band who have sold more than 75 million albums worldwide. Highlights in recent Scorpions years with James include a collaborative album with the Berlin Philharmonic called *Moment Of Glory*, a live unplugged album named *Acoustica* and a live DVD titled *1 Night In Vienna*. Their latest album, *Humanity: Hour 1*, released in 2007, entered the Billboard charts at number 63 and their two-and-a-half-year world tour took them through arenas as far afield as India and South Korea. The band released their latest studio album, *Sting In The Tail*, in 2010.

JESSE HUGHES (b 1972)

Jesse is the enthusiastic frontman of the California-based garage rock band Eagles of Death Metal that he formed in 1998 with high school pal Josh Homme of Kyuss and Queens of the Stone Age fame. When the band finally released their debut album, *Peace, Love, Death Metal,* in 2004, several songs were used in television commercials and video games, including the first single, 'I Only Want You'. Jesse soon fell into a serious drug addiction, later crediting Homme with saving his life. The band's second album, *Death By Sexy,* included backing vocals from Jack Black, who also cameoed with Dave Grohl in the video for first single, 'I Want You So Hard'. The album broke into the *Billboard* 200 and reached number 11 on the Top Independent Albums chart, as they toured with The Strokes and headlined their own US tour. The band received a poor reaction during their first concert as support on the Guns N' Roses 2006 tour, prompting Axl Rose to famously call them the "Pigeons of Shit Metal" on stage – a phrase now tattooed on Jesse's forearm. Their next album, *Heart On,* from 2008 reached number 57 on the charts, propelled by first single, 'Wannabe in L.A.'. The Eagles of Death Metal continue to headline tours in the US and abroad.

JIMMY ASHHURST (b 1963)

Italian-born Jimmy Ashhurst was first introduced to the recording studio when he was taken under the wing of Rat Scabies of seminal UK punk band The Damned. A decade later when Izzy Stradlin quit Guns N' Roses, he chose Jimmy to play bass and tour the world with him in his new outfit, The Ju Ju Hounds. After spending a couple of years in jail due to drug convictions, Jimmy resurrected his music career and joined the hard rock band Buckcherry from Los Angeles. Their next release, entitled *15*, heralded the band's own resurgence with the album going platinum and the multi-platinum hit single 'Crazy Bitch' being nominated for a Grammy. The album also featured the band's first *Billboard* Hot 100 Top 10 hit, 'Sorry'. Dubbed the 'Next Great American Rock Band', Buckcherry's latest album, *Black Butterfly,* debuted in *Billboard*'s Top 10 and was named the iTunes Rock Album of the Year for 2008. The band embarked on a North American tour with Kiss in 2009 and released their first live album, *Live & Loud 2009*. Jimmy continues to enjoy meeting ladies as he tours all around the world with Buckcherry.

JOEL O'KEEFFE (b 1982)

Joel is the young, energetic lead singer and lead guitarist of Airbourne, an Australian pub rock band formed in 2003 in rural Victoria. On the back of an independent EP release in 2004, Capitol Records soon outbid many international labels to sign the band to a multi-million-dollar, five-album worldwide deal, believed to be the largest ever for a never-before-signed Australian band. Airbourne's rowdy and infectious live shows won them support slots for The Rolling Stones, Mötley Crüe and Motörhead, while a main stage place on the Big Day Out festival confirmed their reputation as one of the country's fastest rising bands. However, two months prior to the release of their debut album, Capitol cancelled their lucrative long-term contract. The four-piece signed a new global deal with Roadrunner Records and *Runnin' Wild* was finally released, then nominated for two ARIA Awards and won a *Metal Hammer* Golden Gods Award for Best Debut Album. The band took their booze-and-sweat-soaked rock'n'roll around the world in 2008, including the US, Japan, Europe and sell-out headlining tours of the UK, while gaining valuable exposure through a slew of video games and the WWE. Airbourne's second album, *No Guts, No Glory*, was released early in 2010, with lots of touring scheduled to coincide. Joel's onstage confidence, charisma and cockiness is rarely seen in a frontman in his early twenties, and is a perfect match to Airbourne's fist-pumping, anthemic tracks, full of double entendrés to ensure rock'n'roll will never die.

LEMMY (b 1945)

Born Ian Fraser Kilmister on Christmas Eve, Lemmy is the gravel-voiced singer and bass guitarist for English rock legends Motörhead. After working as a roadie for The Jimi Hendrix Experience in the late Sixties, Lemmy spent four years playing with space rock band Hawkwind, until he was fired in 1975 and spent five days in prison on drugs charges. He then formed the power-trio Motörhead and earned particular success in the early Eighties with a number of UK Top 40 hits, including the classic single 'Ace Of Spades' and the number one live album *No Sleep 'til Hammersmith*. Motörhead won their first Grammy in the awards of 2005 in the Best Metal Performance category. Over their 30-plus-year career, which continues with more albums and world tours today, Motörhead have unquestionably become one of the most influential rock'n'roll bands of all time, and the cool, bona fide bad-ass Lemmy revered as the Godfather of Metal. His instantly recognisable appearance, including facial moles and mutton chops, has even been immortalised with production of an official six-inch action figure. Lemmy is synonymous with the rock'n'roll lifestyle, as supported by his 2002 autobiography, *White Line Fever*. He also landed in the top ten of *Maxim* magazine's 2006 Living Sex Legends list, purporting he has slept with at least 1,200 women.

NICKE BORG (b 1973)

Nicke has been the lead singer and guitarist for Swedish rock band Backyard Babies since 1989. Soon after their debut album, *Diesel & Power,* was released in 1994, the band went on hiatus while guitarist Dregen formed The Hellacopters. However, Dregen returned in 1997 for the band's critically acclaimed album *Total 13* and they've not looked back since, releasing a further four studio albums and touring the world many times over with the likes of Motörhead, AC/DC, Alice Cooper and Social Distortion. The *Making Enemies Is Good* album brought their most commercial success, while the follow-up, *Stockholm Syndrome,* won them a Swedish Grammy award. Their latest album, simply self-titled as *Backyard Babies*, debuted in Sweden at number one on the charts. The band again toured the globe to support the album, playing their lovable brand of booze-fuelled, punk-infused, gutter rock'n'roll that's now earned the quartet worldwide acclaim. Backyard Babies embarked upon a 20th anniversary tour early in 2010 before taking some time out to catch their breath.

ROB PATTERSON (b 1970)

Rob is an American guitarist whose first major band was the hard rock/nu-metal group Otep. They were signed in 2001 after only four shows in LA, without a demo, purely on their powerful and poetic live performances and outspoken political views. Sharon Osbourne was so impressed she offered the unsigned act a slot on the 2001 Ozzfest tour. Their 2002 debut, *Sevas Tra,* reached number 145 on the *Billboard* 200, while their follow-up, *House Of Secrets,* debuted at number 93 two years later. Otep's video for 'Warhead' made the top ten videos of 2004 on MTV's *Headbanger's Ball* as the band toured relentlessly. Rob then began playing guitar for Korn in 2005, starting off with a European tour and culminating with a televised acoustic performance and album, *MTV Unplugged: Korn*. Released worldwide in March 2007, the live album debuted on the *Billboard* 200 at number nine after selling more than 50,000 copies in the US that week. Since departing Korn in 2008, Rob has been working on a full-length solo album, DJ-ing across America (including the Hard Rock Hotel in

Florida and two VMA parties in LA), and working with Otep again on their next album. He is currently engaged to Carmen Electra, the actress-model-dancer sex symbol, famous for her appearances on the TV series *Baywatch* and in *Playboy* magazine.

TOBY RAND (b 1977)

Toby is an Australian rock singer best known for his appearance on the *Rock Star: Supernova* reality television show, which was broadcast to millions worldwide in 2006 as he attempted to become the lead vocalist for a newly formed supergroup featuring Mötley Crüe drummer Tommy Lee, former Metallica bassist Jason Newsted, and former Guns N' Roses guitarist Gilby Clarke. Earning the most encore performances of the contestants, he came third in the show's finale. This helped bring fame to his own band, Juke Kartel, who then toured arenas across North America with Rock Star Supernova and now continue to impress live audiences with performances at premiere events like Australia's MTV Video Awards, Rugby League's World Cup and the Australian F1 Grand Prix. Ever the ladies' man, Toby was also a finalist in *Australian Cleo's* Bachelor of the Year 2008. Juke Kartel toured far and wide in support of their debut album, *Nowhere Left To Hide,* released early in 2009. This included a performance in front of 30,000 people in Norway at Quartz Music Festival before the band relocated to Los Angeles.

VAZQUEZ (b 1976)

Vazquez is the bassist and all-round stud in Damone, an American rock band hailing from Waltham, a city located just west of Boston, Massachusetts. Damone landed their first major record deal with RCA in 2002 and blazed onto the scene with their debut release, *From The Attic*. They quickly found themselves touring all over North America, even having Butch Walker come out and cover a Lita Ford song with them on stage each night during one leg. They worked their way up to the main stage of the Warped festival and toured Japan before releasing their second album, *Out Here All Night*. The album again saw them touring around the US and Japan, plus a couple of tours around the UK. Their music has been featured in several video games, including *Madden NFL 07*, *Project Gotham Racing 2* and *Tony Hawk's Downhill Jam*. The band's songs have also been included in numerous movies and TV shows, while their song 'Revolution' is the official anthem for the New England Revolution of Major League Soccer. Damone's third album, *Roll The Dice*, features the lead vocal debut of Vazquez on the song 'Talk Of The Town', which is accompanied by a raunchy promotional video.

BEAUTY & ATTRACTION

"GIRLS WHO FUCK ROCK STARS KNOW HOW TO DO IT WITH THEIR EYES"

What do you find to be most attractive in a sexual partner?

ACEY SLADE: Confidence, for sure. But if a girl's too aggressive or too easy, then that's totally a turn-off. I think it's important sometimes to make the distinction between what's sex and what's looking for something that's going to go somewhere. Of course the first part is sexual attraction because nobody wants to be in a long-term relationship with someone they're not sexually attracted to – I hope. So, in general, aesthetics, but personality-wise, confidence and they have to have a sense of humour.

ADDE: The thing is that I always kind of like manly-looking girls for some reason, and they kind of like me for looking like a manly chick. I like hands; I'm not much of an ass person or a tit person. I look at hands and I really get off on hands… and if I can see the veins and stuff. I kind of like manly hands. I get off on that… and I'm totally straight!

ALLISON ROBERTSON: Probably if they're bigger than I am. I'm relatively petite but I'm not necessarily attracted when a guy is smaller or skinnier than me, which exits out a lot of rock'n'rollers because they're all so skinny and praying mantis-like. I like when guys are big and strong. Also, it's really generic as girls say it all the time, but I think when you have a little bit more of a brain you can appreciate someone who is really funny. Not just goofy funny. I need somebody that can really make me laugh because I don't really laugh out loud that much at comedy unless it's a little edgy. We've seen a lot of stuff travelling and in my band especially, there's not much we haven't seen in the way of comedy. So a guy that's a little funnier than the rest turns me on. I think it's really sexy.

BLASKO: For me personally, I definitely like dark hair. I definitely like big tits and I like a good smile too, and a good laugh – that's really attractive to me. I definitely also like something exotic too; I'm not overly attracted to someone plain. I like a little bit of exoticness, whether that be like Asian or Latino… Spanish of some kind.

BRUCE KULICK: There's certainly something about a girl's eyes. If a girl has a great figure, she has an amazing rack and a great ass that's all great, but if they're kind of fugly (as we say) that's taking away something. There's always something about that connection of looking into a girl's eyes. As much as I'm as horny as the next guy, as to like 'Oh, she's got a smokin' body', I also want to have some kind of connection and when you look at a girl's eyes, that's how you connect. So for me, there's always something about when I look into their eyes; obviously I've already scoped out everything else in the first nanosecond. I've been attracted to some women in my life where you can tell they're really troubled and they can't even really make eye contact, and I'm like, 'OK, that's a hot chick but I'm not going to connect with that'. I want to feel like I'm comfortable with the person, so that's why I need that connection. I need to be able to look in their eyes and they should be showing me attraction and they should be accepting my affection; then I can take it to the next level.

CHIP Z'NUFF: The first thing to catch me is the person's disposition, how they carry themselves. Playing in a rock band, you have plenty of opportunity to meet people. It's a great occupation for meeting the opposite sex. However, you know right away when you meet somebody if they trip your trigger or not.

COURTNEY TAYLOR-TAYLOR: I think what attracts our eye is pretty much proven to be the same for everyone: a certain amount of space between the eyes and cheekbone with the mouth. They're all pretty standard things. For me to specifically pick out somebody, it's got to have a lot to do with the way their body moves around. Like, is it confident, is it cautious? It's about the balance of psychologies that are apparent in body languages and body motion. I'm pretty clinical about it too. I really believe it is all just maths and science that attracts us to people. When I was younger, I thought it was just straight-up clothes and haircut – any relatively healthy female with the right clothes and haircut, and that's partially right. That's partially true because that is how we broadcast what we care about and what we want in this life, visually, without having to have a conversation, without even having to be within ten feet of somebody. With every decision we make about how we dress, we're broadcasting who we are, who we want to be, who we hope to be, who we want to be with, who we want our friends to be, who we want to fit in with. So when I first thought about it, I wanted a girl to look and seem like they listened to The Buzzcocks and read Ayn Rand. I went through a lot of different things and something I never thought I would really be attracted to is someone who's just really fucking nice, who isn't acting nice until they get in all the way into your life and your heart and your days and nights, and then they just start showing that they're actually mean and condescending.

DANKO JONES: I have to be honest: she's got to be hot! For me at least, she's got to be very pretty and she's got to have a great body. But that's not a deal-breaker. The deal-breaker would be if she's insecure and very needy. That's pretty much a deal-breaker, no matter how hot she is. That tells me that she won't be able to handle weeks and sometimes months away from home while I'm out on the road. That's always been a deal-breaker for me: if a girl, no matter how hot she is, is very needy and very insecure with herself. It's a trait that over the years has become very important to me.

DOUG ROBB: The first thing that comes to my mind is confidence, to be honest with you. Right after that, it's face. I think you can have a drop-dead, gorgeous body and a beautiful face but if you're very intimidated and shy and insecure for whatever reasons, it's a definite turn-off. If you have what you consider an average face or not the best body or whatever and you exude that type of confidence, there's something extremely sexy about that.

EVAN SEINFELD: I'll say for sure it's an intangible, indescribable air of pheromonal sexual confidence. I like women who know what they want and who aren't pretending. I find so many women are not really interested in sex, only what they can get *from* the sex – where men are more interested in sex *for* the sex. I like girls who are physically fit; I love a flat stomach on a girl. I love a round, high-up bottom that you can bounce a quarter off. I love tits of all sizes, but whether they're big or small they've got to defy gravity.

WITH BIG BOOBS COMES A CONFIDENT WOMAN AND I LIKE CONFIDENCE IN WOMEN. I LIKE A WOMAN WITH CONFIDENCE AND BIG BOOBS.

HANDSOME DICK MANITOBA: My first answer is tits and ass; that's the first thing that comes to my mind. But it all has to start with step one, which is that look in the eye. It's that look in the eye when you realise you're connecting. It could be born out of sitting and talking to someone, where all of a sudden you realise, 'Holy shit! I am connecting!' That's like the hottest thing in the world because what that does… you can't put the food on the table before you have a nice tablecloth – that's the tablecloth.

JAMES KOTTAK: Hair – it has to be blonde. And I must say I like big boobs. With big boobs comes a confident woman and I like confidence in women. I like a woman with confidence and big boobs.

JESSE HUGHES: Attractive is definitely an eye of the beholder thing, so to speak. Some people find tits attractive and that's why some women get boob jobs, which is a damn shame. Some dudes find easiness attractive more so than other things. It depends on my mood. If I'm walking the bookstore circuit at night, I'm definitely a different animal. I like someone who when you whisper something dirty to them they smile but they look around to make sure no one else heard.

JIMMY ASHHURST: I tend to regard the whole package, but hygiene rates highly on that list and I'm a big legs and ass guy.

JOEL O'KEEFFE: Her sexual desire and how much she lets it show. Girls that get flirty and talk a little dirty right from the get-go always get my undivided attention, as it's a guarantee that once we're alone, I'll have a lot of fun burying my bone.

LEMMY: Beauty is in the eye of the beholder as we all know. It seems a cliché but it's still true. I've seen people with people that you can't believe. You see this ravishing chick with this spotty geezer with glasses and you think, 'Why? He hasn't got any money.' It really is in the eye of the beholder. You can never tell. To me, I'm a legs and breasts man.

NICKE BORG: I think understanding. First of all, I think a person that actually falls for you for looks or the person that you are, without knowing that you are actually in a band. And also a person that maybe knows you're in a band, but kind of understands that being in a band is sometimes very lonely and tragic, and they understand that. It's not all like, 'I want to fuck you to pieces because I've seen your video man.'

ROB PATTERSON: Brains, sexual essence, and ass – got to have a bangin' ass!

TOBY RAND: Confidence: for instance, that may mean that if a girl walks into a room, she is immediately seen and is known. You know she's there; she's present, and with that comes a positive attitude, smile… and a really good ass.

VAZQUEZ: I really look for a voluptuous woman. I want a big ass; I want big tits. Skinny girls – they're just no fun. Like, it just doesn't feel good. I want a woman that feels like a woman.

What's the best way for someone to snare a rock star millionaire?

EVAN SEINFELD: It's all in the eyes – the unspoken language. Girls who fuck rock stars know how to do it with their eyes. Sometimes I could look out in the crowd when I'm performing and our eyes could meet and sometimes I don't even have to have sex with them because we already had, you know.

JIMMY ASHHURST: It seems to me that Los Angeles has become the Mecca for that sort of a girl. Every club is quite full up with that variety. They're quick enough to check the fuckin' *Billboard* charts before they'll go out with you. They'll do a background check on your credit report as well. It's become a viable sort of career choice these days. It seems it's not quite as rebellious as it used to be: back in the day, if a girl was to snare a millionaire rock star husband there'd be plenty of bullshit she'd have to 'pay for' during the relationship, but now it seems like the guys that they're after are a calmer, more reasonable sort.

JOEL O'KEEFFE: Probably the same as with anyone: just get them crazy drunk, or high.

ROB PATTERSON: I wouldn't know but from what I hear, don't stalk! Be yourself!

TOBY RAND: It's to be confident and to treat them exactly the same way you would treat anyone else. They're not bigger than anyone else.

VAZQUEZ: All you have to do is just kind of be yourself. Sometimes you'll see a girl at a show and she'll meet you and go 'Hi' and then there's nothing – she's shy and that doesn't work. She doesn't have to be super forward, but just enough.

Do blondes really have more fun?

ACEY SLADE: Nah.

ADDE: Probably, probably. I've known a lot of blonde women who've especially had a lot of fun. Maybe that's like a female thing. I don't know if that applies to men.

ALLISON ROBERTSON: Well I was born with pretty light-coloured hair and as I turned older it turned brown and I became much shyer. The second that my hair turned brown I became a nerd… I'm just kidding. But really it happens to a lot of people where they're born with light hair and it gets dark. To be honest, I always dyed my hair darker than it actually is. It's like a golden colour and the last two years it's been blonde and I've got to say it does kind of let the wild child out a little more than I was expecting. I bleached it in high school before and it was really short and stuff, but I have to say you do feel a little more sex kitten-like with the bleached blonde hair. Also, I asked for my hairdresser to leave in the roots and I wanted it to be really messy like David Lee Roth. There is something about it when you can just roll the windows down and cruise around Hollywood with the blonde hair flowing. You do feel pretty sexy. It does kind of seem fun. I do think it attracts people that are looking for fun as well. People zero-in on you like, 'Hey, she looks fun!'

ANDREW W.K.: I don't know if they have more fun, but a natural blonde woman is very pretty. I was with a girl that was naturally blonde and I was so excited that I was going to get to be with this blonde girl because I'd never been with a blonde girl before; it had always been a brown-haired girl. I think this was like the second or third girl I'd ever been with intimately. It was before I started touring. I was living in New York and I was just getting my Andrew W.K. act going and just developing new levels of confidence. I was so excited that I was going to be with a blonde-haired girl, not just about does the carpet match the drapes but like, she had fair skin, her eyes were blue, she had blonde hair and it was really new. Of course, the day we went on our first date after having hung out a lot, she shows up and she had dyed her hair brown! It was such a bummer. I couldn't help but say, 'Wow, you look great but I'm a little disappointed. I was so excited about you with your blonde hair.' I had a crush on a girl in high school who was just beautiful. I had a crush on her for a couple of years; she was in the older grade than me and she had blonde hair. The whole face of a person looks different when they have blonde hair, especially when it's a natural blonde; again, the colouring is entirely different.

BRENT MUSCAT: No, I don't think so. I've dated blondes before but I think I prefer darker-haired girls, brunettes and stuff. What's attractive to me though is a woman who's open-minded. Someone you can take to dinner and they're at least willing to try different types of food, and just be open-minded about stuff. Some of my girlfriends in the past would probably be considered not very attractive, but that's not the most important thing to me. Apart from just looks, I think I need to have a bit of a deeper connection.

BRUCE KULICK: You know, it's funny: I'm dark-haired and brown-eyed and I'm definitely attracted to blondes and blue eyes, and others. I've been really attracted to Latino women and Asian women – I'll just say women! For a while there, Cindy Crawford did it for me and that's totally not your typical blonde chick. Some of my favourites were always like Heather Graham; and she almost kind of does look like she could live next door to you. Pamela Anderson I think is awfully hot and that's why it always blew me away with Tommy [Lee] and Kid Rock having their fun with her, but I wouldn't last a minute in her presence. I wouldn't be able to form a sentence; I couldn't really relax. I need more of a girl-next-door. But is she hot and off the scale? Of course, but I wouldn't survive that. But again, for me in many ways, it's the connection and beauty in the eyes. As much as a blonde is always my favourite, I've certainly been lustful for women who are not blonde.

CHIP Z'NUFF: It's just a rumour. It's been circulating for years. I think maybe after you change your look you might feel like there are better things happening because your whole disposition changes, so maybe in some ways it's true, but for the most part I think it's just an old fallacy.

COURTNEY TAYLOR-TAYLOR: They probably have more fun than goths but probably not as much fun as curly redheads.

DANKO JONES: I am partial to that hair colour, yes.

DOUG ROBB: I don't think so. I was actually talking to my wife about this a few days ago because I think most of the girls I've dated in my life have been blonde but it's never been like I prefer blondes; I never have. I always kind of go for the face and whatever hair colour they have after that is insignificant. I don't think they necessarily have more fun.

EVAN SEINFELD: Blondes definitely do not have more fun. I love blondes but I'm definitely a brunette man first. My first preference is Asian and Eurasian, my second preference is Latin, my third preference is brunette and my fourth preference is blonde. I've had sex with women of every ethnicity imaginable, different races and nationalities, and I do find that girls who are blonde but not naturally blonde – what I call bottle blondes – are usually the most insecure and really enjoy it the least. They're doing it out of emptiness, loneliness and desperation. One thing that turns me off is girls who are fucking out of trying to make themselves feel better about themselves rather than trying to enjoy themselves. That's not to say it's an absolute rule, just my personal experience thing.

HANDSOME DICK MANITOBA: I have no idea. Everyone in my family has brown eyes and brown hair. I've gone out with very few blondes in my life. I'm a New York Jew, as you might or might not know, and the unobtainable goddesses like Claudia Schiffer, the blonde, blue-eyed Aryan beauties that we all sort of pine for, are actually not my favourite type of girl. My favourite type of girl is more of the Adriana Lima, Mediterranean, olive skin or dark skin with dark eyes and dark hair. So blondes might have more fun, but those smouldering brunettes are the way to go.

JAMES KOTTAK: Absolutely, of course they do! It's true, it's true!

JESSE HUGHES: Oh hell no! Oh God no! Blondes are golden; that's what makes them special. They're golden and therefore they're coveted often, but do they have more fun? Oh hell no, I'll tell you that right now! Brunettes look like hot secretaries and the mother of your good friend who you love to see when you go over to his house on pool day.

JIMMY ASHHURST: Blondes are definitely more of a bash-you-over-the-head sort, like 'Here I am!' Being an equal opportunity employer though, I find something smouldering in the brunettes; I do like those. But on the surface, I think blondes definitely have more fun.

JOEL O'KEEFFE: Blondes, natural or dyed, are my true weakness. I've crashed my car three times checking them out and spent all my money taking them out, but once you reel them in and get them alone, they're always worth it. Blondes, again natural or dyed, automatically know they're sexy, so I would have to say blondes *do* have more fun. They scream louder, they cum harder, they go harder, they're always wet and horny as hell, and when you think it's over, they're always ready for another round.

LEMMY: I don't know; I've never been blonde.

NICKE BORG: Yeah, dude. I'm blonde. Even though I shave, I'm fucking blonde.

ROB PATTERSON: That depends. In my case, yes.

TOBY RAND: No, no they don't. Black-haired girls have more fun... Any girl has fun. It doesn't matter what colour hair they have 'cause a lot of blondes actually do have black hair.

VAZQUEZ: Hmmm... I'm going through the Rolodex in my mind – I think fake blondes have more fun.

Are tattoos and piercings turn-ons for rock stars? What regions are sexiest?

ACEY SLADE: It's kind of become predictable now and it's probably rare that you find a girl, especially a groupie, that doesn't have any tattoos or piercings. I like a girl who looks very clean on the face and on the hands and is maybe wearing a sweater. She takes off the sweater and she's got maybe a sleeve or a cool back-piece.

ADDE: I guess it is... doesn't really matter, really.

ALLISON ROBERTSON: I've got to say with tattoos, I think they can be really sexy but they have to be smart. I get really turned-off when it's bad tattoos. It's all in your taste and everybody's got different taste levels in what they like. For me, stuff like tribal tattoos is not really my style or when people have Chinese characters and they don't even... I actually took Japanese so I know what some of the kanji means. So sometimes I'm like, 'Do you even know what that means?' and they're like, 'Oh, I think it means like I'm relaxed' and it doesn't even mean that at all; it means tree or I'm going to pee on your house or something. I think tattoos are only sexy when they actually mean something, like when you can tell somebody's travelled a lot. I think it's cool when people get tattoos, like guys in bands or girls in bands, and they've collected them like you would stickers when you were a kid or something; like stamps, they're from all different places all over the world, all that shit. I think it's much sexier when it comes from somewhere, as opposed to just trying to look cool. Piercings: to be honest, I've never even dated somebody that has a piercing. Maybe a one-ear piercing that closed up a long time ago. It's not a turn-off necessarily, but I've never really gone that route with guys.

ANDREW W.K.: I've never liked them unto themselves, so I wouldn't be more attracted to a girl that had piercings or tattoos. There's definitely been times where, not that I had been turned-off specifically by tattoos or piercings, but sometimes the girl that has had a lot of tattoos and piercings also had other vibes about them (that maybe inspired them to get those tattoos and piercings) that didn't gel too well with me. I don't think it was the tattoos and piercings themselves. I'm very happy now that my wife only has her ears pierced and no tattoos. I think it's amazing because there are so many girls who have tattoos. I think tattoos are cool. I have tattoos but they're just designs. There's something about just looking at pictures all day that to me is pretty intense. It's just like if you're in your house and you have some paintings on your wall; if you're going to walk by those paintings every day for 50 years, you'd better really like those paintings and often at times I bet you'll feel like taking them down and moving them or changing things a bit so you don't see the same atmosphere, you don't have the same decoration. So decorating your body with paintings and pictures is really intense, but I admire people that do it. I think it's great. I have my ears pierced. I used to want my nose pierced and things like that. If I was looking at naked pictures of a girl for example, I would prefer that she had no piercings or tattoos.

PIERCED TONGUES ARE TOTALLY, TOTALLY IRRITATING BECAUSE THEY GENERALLY SPEND THE MAJORITY OF THEIR TIME CLACKING THAT THING AGAINST THEIR TEETH

BLASKO: Pierced nipples are really cool, but that's about the end of it for me. Pierced tongues are totally, totally irritating because they generally spend the majority of their time clacking that thing against their teeth – it's like nails on a chalkboard to me. So pierced nipples are great and tattoos I don't mind so much but it kind of depends on what it is. I think there's a fine line between a piece that was done well and had some thought put behind it, versus like 'Fuck you' or something on their shoulder, which I've seen.

BRENT MUSCAT: I think a belly pierced is kind of sexy. I'm not super into full-sleeve tattoos on girls, or a lot of facial tattoos. Something like on the back, nicely placed, is fine but that's not to say I prefer tattoos. Either way I think, so long as they're attractive. I think the worst is when a girl has a prison-look tattoo. I don't think that's attractive, or the chest plate tattoo that some girls are now getting. I don't really find that attractive. I like something that can be kind of hidden and if it's revealed in the bedroom then that's a little sexier I'd say. It's funny: I've made it through all these years of rock'n'roll and I don't have one tattoo.

BRUCE KULICK:
Probably for your average rock star who already has tattoos and all, they probably think it's awesome. It's not like it's completely horrible to me but it's not a turn-on at all for me. If they have a few in tasteful spots, I'm OK with it. If they're completely tattooed, they probably won't even be attracted to me because I don't represent that. I have one ear pierced; that's it. I have friends that absolutely think I am a great guy, guitar player, musician, friend who are completely sleeved (I'm talking about guys and girls), but I don't think I would be in a relationship at any time with a girl that was heavily tattooed. I could see maybe one or two but... Again, it's very rock'n'roll and it's very now. You can't deny the fashion of it, shall I say, but I'm a little old-fashioned about that. Even though Angelina Jolie is a great actress and I think she's beautiful, the stuff that's all over her body, I don't get it – I just don't get it. She's not a musician or a rocker or anything and I'm still going like, 'What?' So I don't know. I can see how some women could do a little nose thing here or... some of them even do something down on their vagina and I'm like, 'What?' I've experienced some of those kinds of things and I'm not saying it was something that completely turned me off but it gave me more of a, 'Wait a minute; this isn't my kind of girl.' The tongue thing too... some of the girls that express themselves that way certainly feel it's a sexual aid to please their man, or their girl, but I couldn't tell you if that's true or not. I haven't had enough experience with that; it's just not something I'm attracted to.

CHIP Z'NUFF:
Well it seems to be that tattoos and piercings are a big part of attraction to rock'n'rollers because most of the dudes have that. However, if you can be somebody that doesn't have that, I think that makes it a little more original. I remember hanging out at A&M Studios in Los Angeles where Enuff Z'Nuff were recording an album and Ozzy Osbourne was in the other room. He wouldn't let anyone in his room. Ozzy had a little sign on his door that said 'Absolutely No Admittance'. So we put a sign on our door that said 'Absolutely No Admittance Unless You Have the Following: Cocaine, Crack, Heroin, Pot, Alcohol, Trim'. I was sitting outside with Ozzy – I finally got a chance to sit down and talk with him, and I love him to death by the way – and he says, 'You want to be original? Don't get a fucking tattoo!' So no tattoos and piercings for me.

COURTNEY TAYLOR-TAYLOR:
Piercings have never been a thing I could relate to, or tolerate, or anything. I guess I liked it when nose rings and the eyebrow ring came into fashion. I thought that was pretty cool; I still do. I really liked it when it went out of fashion so that those people who had that thing that I actually think looks kind of cool still had that and were actually making it a rather individualist statement, ten years later, again. Any kind of nipple rings or any kind

of genital piercing stuff to me is just sad. Like, 'Oh, I always thought you were so cool but now you're a mess. You've got problems – a lot of them – and you're just sad; a sad person.' That's what that shit says to me now; it always has since the first time I saw nipple rings or a Prince Albert. I don't like the lower-back tattoo exposed either.

DANKO JONES: I know guys sway either way, like some guys think that a lot of tattoos on a girl is very attractive and I know guys who really get turned-on by girls who have sleeves. It doesn't really come into play with me. After the looks thing, it's more of a personality. Tattoos don't decide whether I'm even going to consider asking her out or anything; it has nothing to do with anything really.

DOUG ROBB: Me personally, I don't think piercings are a turn-on. Tattoos can be cool, especially legitimate tattoos, like maybe a girl who has a quarter-sleeve or a sleeve, or something like that. Or tattoos around the front of the hips and stuff like that; that's cool. The typical small-of-the-back fairy or tribal armband is definitely not sexy. In fact, if this is Sex Tips from the Rock Stars, I think nowadays if you don't have any tattoos you're more rock'n'roll than if you do. Having tattoos used to be a symbol of your rebelliousness I guess, but now honestly, besides myself and our guitar player, I don't know who the fuck doesn't have tattoos – everybody does! We're like the last of the dying breed.

EVAN SEINFELD: I think a lot of women think that just because rock stars are personally tattooed or pierced that we want them to be tattooed as well. I'm very selective how I feel about that. I've got to say that I'm not a fan of tattooed women as much as I am of girls with little or no tattoos. If a girl's going to have a tattoo, to me they've got to have quality tattoos. I don't like when girls have tattoos that I would have; it makes them look kind of manly. They don't need any lower-back tramp stamps; definitely don't need any breast tattoos in between the tits, ladies. I hate coloured tattoos on anybody. What's sexy to me is a girl with a small tattoo on her neck, or a small tattoo on her finger, or behind her ear. Piercings: I'm a big fan lately of that kind of Marilyn Monroe little dot on the cheek called a Monroe I think; I like that. I personally think like one piercing on a girl; she could have like a labret or a septum, or a tiny little nose ring, but once you put multiple piercings, to me it's almost distracting. In this pop culture where every fucking basketball player, football player, rapper... where tattoos have kind of crossed over into the norms of mainstream pop culture, I think that a lot of women see it like a rock'n'roll mating call, like a tribal thing where, 'Hey I've got tattoos, you've got tattoos, we've got tattoos together.' Not to say I don't sleep with girls with tattoos but I will definitely say it's not my first preference.

GINGER: I don't think tattoos or piercings make any difference either way. Aside from the initial 'she's cute', it's the person's compatibility that makes any relationship work. Once you've established a common attraction then consistency is the main glue to any successful relationship.

HANDSOME DICK MANITOBA: Basically, I'm not a big fan at all, as a turn-on, but I've got to deal with the reality of the world around me. I deal with it. My wife has just got her whole arm tattooed and I bought it for her as a present. Part of being in a relationship is the art of compromise; the art of acceptance. You can be sexual all you want but that day-to-day, fibrous material that relationships are made from is about acceptance of other people and compromise.

JAMES KOTTAK: I'm totally into tattoos. I'm not into man tattoos on women. I like the odd tattoo here and there. I don't care for the sleeves on chicks. Piercings on the face – got to go. I don't dig it. So I think it's really sexy when a girl has girly tattoos; I love that.

JESSE HUGHES: They're turn-ons for anyone who's horny. Genuinely, rock stars are what they are because they're really horny, however you want to dress it up. You can pretend it's about art or saving whales or some shit like that, but it's always about someone being real horny. I think piercings can be rad, unless of course it's a piercing that looks like they're about to cut your dick in half or something that says you're really not going to enjoy everything that's about to happen. Everything that a person wears on their body is a message and sometimes you've got to pick it up.

JIMMY ASHHURST: I'm not one to particularly go out of my way to look for that sort of thing. I tend to like the ones who also have… jobs. So whether it is acting or modelling or whatever; those are the ones who seldom have too many piercings.

JOEL O'KEEFFE: Ink and steel is sexy as hell! It's always a welcome surprise when you're ripping each other's clothes off and you discover a cool piece of art, or your tongue touches that little piece of warm, wet steel. It's like finding buried treasure and you've got it all to yourself.

NICKE BORG: It's totally unique from person to person I think. There's nothing sexier than an innocent girl who doesn't even know what a tattoo or piercing is basically. But there's nothing more of a turn-off than having a little dolphin on their shoulder. A really, really big dragon or a skull tattooed all over the fucking back on a girl is cool. Like, you don't really see that in the first place. They're walking around in a little skirt, and then you're like, 'Woah, shit!' So it depends; it's a case-by-case basis. Tattoos are a bit sexual in a way, but I wouldn't go for the dolphin or a little bunny on the shoulder.

ROB PATTERSON: Yes. For me, not totally covered but in certain places like behind the ear, wrists… nothing too extreme.

TOBY RAND: I think tattoos are extremely sexy and I think the best region for girls would be the nape of their neck, on their wrists, on their ankles, and just leading towards their pelvic area.

VAZQUEZ: I love nipple rings. I'm not really crazy about all the genital piercings and shit like that. The other piercing I really don't like on girls (or even on guys too) is when they stretch out their ear lobe. I remember being at this show and I was talking to a girl. It was loud and I got close and it just smelled and I was like, 'Eeeewww, what the fuck is that? This is gross!' Ears are made that way – you don't need to fuck with them.

Do rock stars go for youth and inexperience, or mature and experienced partners?

ACEY SLADE: I'd take mature and experienced any day. You play with babies, you clean up diapers.

ALLISON ROBERTSON: I guess it depends what you're looking for but I personally prefer someone who's a little bit more experienced and is a lot more mature. Because you're in a band, you go for other people in bands or in the music industry, but people don't grow up right when they're on tour all the time. They don't do the same things as someone who's been at home and gone to school and got a bunch of crappy jobs. When you date someone who's only ever had a bunch of girls and never had a real girlfriend, and vice versa, they don't really know what they're doing sometimes. They're kind of just used to being pleased and they don't know how to make it go back and forth. So I am much more partial to someone who's hopefully a little bit older than I am; age doesn't really matter but the maturity level does, totally.

BLASKO: Mature and experienced.

CHIP Z'NUFF: Mature and experienced, absolutely. Youth and inexperience only can go so far but there's nothing like having knowledge. Knowledge is everything, as my grandfather would say. With knowledge, there is nothing that will stop you, except for yourself.

DANKO JONES: Ideally it would be great if she was younger than me and had the experience. That's my ideal. I don't really enjoy being a teacher. When I was a kid, the whole thing about having a virgin was the ultimate fantasy for men. When I grew up and started becoming sexually active, I realised very quickly that that's a turn-off. It's a real turn-off to be with a woman who's inexperienced. I don't find the whole virgin fantasy my type of fantasy. I really enjoy being with a woman who knows what she wants in bed and that comes through experience; she's very secure with herself in bed, knows what she wants, and is very good at it.

EVAN SEINFELD: I think that depends on the time and the place. In other words, if it's Wednesday night and we're playing in Slovakia and the tour bus is leaving in two hours, I've got no time to educate somebody. I definitely want a girl who... she doesn't have to be experienced but at least a girl who knows what she wants. There are so many girls who are so conflicted about what they want to do. A lot of girls are just looking for attention and I'd like to put it out there: don't waste our time ladies. We don't really want to be your friend; we don't really want to talk to you. Most of us have a wife or a girlfriend at home that we want to spend our quality time with. So, if you want sex, let us know. If you don't, there should be a law against false advertising! There should be like liquidated damages clauses.

There is something really sexy about a youthful, inexperienced girl. Part of the series that I'm actually performing sex in for a new company Tera and I have called Iron Cross – if you go to rockstarpimp.com you can see that I have different series for smoking-hot brunettes, smoking-hot blondes, smoking-hot Asians, smoking-hot Latinos... and two of my favourites are smoking-hot thinners, which are girls who weigh 105 or less, and then smoking-hot teens. There's something very sexy about it; that age of innocence. To me, by the time a lot of girls have been around a few times and they get a little older, even as early as their late twenties, a lot of girls are really screwed up because they've been fucked over by a boyfriend or two and they become jaded; it becomes really obvious. And there's something really sexy about the innocence of a girl who just wants to experience it; I'm really turned on by that. When my wife and I discuss the kind of girls I'm going to have sex with on film, she always tells me, 'Evan, get the hottest, youngest girls you can find because they're not fucked up yet.' My wife is an expert on that shit; she's the queen of all hot chicks.

HANDSOME DICK MANITOBA: I hate to answer a simple sounding question with a detailed answer but when you ask, 'Do you go for…' well, I'm a man. I'm a caveman. Cavemen never vary and never really evolved so… I don't want to sound like a pervert, even at 55, but if I'm watching a teenage show with my six-year-old son and I see a 16-year-old girl, it's a cute 16-year-old girl! I don't sit back and go, 'I'm 55. I can't think she's cute.' If I were out having a one night stand, I'd go for anything that turned me on. If I were looking for a mate, as just arm candy, three days I'd be bored out of my mind. So when you say, 'What would you look for,' I have to preface it with that. If I was a bachelor, I would go with whatever felt good at that moment. Like a fly towards the light (which eventually kills them). But if I was looking for someone I could hang out with and spend time with and go to level B, C and D of a relationship with, I'd have to have somebody a little older.

JIMMY ASHHURST: I personally prefer youth and inexperienced. I think experience is highly over-rated.

JOEL O'KEEFFE: These days the youth are experienced and the experienced stay fit and youthful, so either one is a winner.

LEMMY: You just go for who you go for, don't you, really? You don't exactly enquire about their background. It isn't the Presidential race. It's just like, if you fancy it, you go for it, don't you?

NICKE BORG: I would say that I think it comes with age; these days it's too much of an effort to go through that, 'Ooh ahh, be gentle.' I'm like, 'Pfff, whatever.' But also when they're like, 'Fuck me in the ass with your cell phone,' I'm like, 'No way dude, I just wanna…,' you know. So I think somewhere in between. It's a turn-on in a way with someone that's not that sexually experienced but it can also be a turn-off going with someone who's shaved and going, 'Shove your head up my pussy' and I'm like, 'No!'

I REALLY ENJOY BEING WITH A WOMAN WHO KNOWS WHAT SHE WANTS IN BED AND THAT COMES THROUGH EXPERIENCE

ROB PATTERSON: Mature and experienced!

TOBY RAND: Initially we go for youth because they're the ones who are energetic and eager to please, but then after we've had the youth, we like maturity.

VAZQUEZ: I think that depends on what you want. I think a little of both is best. Like, not so experienced that it's like a business transaction. I remember this one time there was this girl who came into the hotel with a dildo in her purse and I'm like, 'C'mon, do you really need to try that hard?' That was a bit much, so I gave her the best 45 seconds I could.

How can someone impress a rock star enough to take the next sexual step?

ACEY SLADE: Oh, that's easy: don't fuck on the first night... Unless you just want to fuck them – then fuck them.

ADDE: What I tend to kind of fall for is not the rock chicks. I tend to fall for those who are, 'No, I'm just here because my friend would like to see you guys. I'm a librarian you know' or something like that. I tend to fall for those kinds of girls. So be as un- rock'n'roll as possible and I will get interested.

JOEL O'KEEFFE: Rock stars are always hungry for love, so just provide them with something enticing to eat and the job's right.

ROB PATTERSON: If you have it, you have it; if you don't, you don't.

TOBY RAND: Lead the way. Tell *me* what to do.

CLOTHING & LINGERIE

"I LIKE THINGS THAT MAKE THE THIGHS AND HINDQUARTERS ENHANCED TO SQUEEZE AND PINCH IN THOSE AREAS WHERE THE FLESH IS REALLY TENDER"

What is the hottest lingerie?

ACEY SLADE: Garter belts for sure, hands-down. And expensive stuff: I like girls who are wearing Agent Provocateur or something like that.

ADDE: The classic… like basically when it comes to women, the classic look. I like them to hide themselves so there's more to reveal; more to take off. Then when they're naked it's like, 'Wow, this is so taboo!' So, the classic stuff – really, really classic.

ALLISON ROBERTSON: I like lace. I know that lots of guys like black lace and stuff, but to me, I'm more into like pastel… To be honest, I'll tell you what: I'm a Virgo (I don't know if it has anything to do with my taste as far as that goes) but I like stuff that looks almost virginal. I like lingerie that almost looks like what you'd wear on your wedding night. Not that I wear that every day but I think I'm partial to white and kind of pristine looking – like 'the good girl' but obviously you're so not good, as opposed to the obvious I'm in a rock band and I wear black all the time. I think it's more interesting when someone doesn't know what you're going to be wearing underneath too. I like having a different character or whatever when wearing lingerie. I also really like the Eighties kind of… like the Mötley Crüe 'Girls, Girls, Girls' video and that Eighties stripper stuff. To me that's really hot lingerie. They still have stuff like that; if you go to a strip club you'll see things like that, but things have changed over the years. I still like it when I see a video like that. I like those kind of bodies on a girl and I think women should be looking more like that, a little voluptuous. To me that's the ultimate look with lingerie: the Eighties stripper look.

ANDREW W.K.: I like garter belts. I like things that make the thighs and hindquarters enhanced to squeeze and pinch in those areas where the flesh is really tender. You can see the lace or the elastic making an imprint and creating an indentation. Lingerie that really creates nice indentations, that's what I'm looking for.

BLASKO: I'm not into lingerie. You know, I like clothes and I like undressing and I like naked, but whatever's naturally underneath the first set of clothes is what I like. But actually taking something off to put something on to take it off again is kind of irritating to me.

BRENT MUSCAT: I like fishnets; I like see-through stuff. Even regular pyjamas are very cute if they're tight or whatever. But I definitely like something see-through and sexy, like a fishnet type of thing.

BRUCE KULICK: For me, and I've always been this way and I certainly express it when I'm in a relationship, I think fishnets are just absolutely awesome on girls. I just think it's the sexiest thing a girl could wear. I have no idea why. Of course it's definitely an important piece of lingerie; it definitely is. But why that one is my favourite in particular, I don't really know. When a girl wants to dress up like a French maid or a school girl, I like that because I like the innocence that turns into, 'Now I'm going to fuck your brains out.' Or the secretary, where the girl has got the hair up and glasses, then that all comes off. All that really works for me; it really does. Your girl who is obviously sexed-out and is slutty and is dressed that way and is acting that way, I'm going to run from. I want a little game, a little mystery. I won't use the word cute, but I want the girl to represent themselves to me, that I have some sort of effect on them, that they're going to entertain me and not be a bimbo. And I think the ways I was describing it, in those kinds of outfits, there's some submissiveness there and coyness that I think is fun. And obviously those are popular outfits on Valentine's Day… and Halloween if a girl wants to do that. I'm not into the horror stuff either and I don't find that a turn-on. I have friends who think that's kind of cool with fangs and blood, but that doesn't do it for me.

CHIP Z'NUFF: I like stuff that's subtle, myself. Although with over-the-top, there are definitely times of the day where that could be exciting. But if I had my choice, it'd be something real subtle. The little things I think catch your attention. Also leaving something to be desired, leaving a little bit there, so that you're not sure exactly what's there, has always been enticing.

COURTNEY TAYLOR-TAYLOR: White cotton anything. Anything without lace – white cotton, loose fitting and not a thong. Actually, I'm going to get more specific here: I'm going to go with low-rise, wide-sides, hip-hugger underwear for girls – white cotton. Then a wifebeater, kind of stretched-out and worn-out, thin and too big.

DANKO JONES: I don't like lingerie. I like a woman who is butt naked. If anything, I like maybe high heels, but that's about it. But high heels in bed are ridiculous! It just doesn't work. It works in *Hustler* magazine. It just doesn't work in real life in bed.

DOUG ROBB: Man, it always changes with the times. I think boy shorts underwear where half your ass is showing is probably the best look; maybe just a short, little, tight T-shirt on top of that. I think that's frickin' hot.

EVAN SEINFELD: My personal favourite lingerie is my wife's line, Mistress Couture. It's her own fucking lingerie brand; it's really sexy, a lot of black, very low-cut. I think it's got to be young; I think it's got to be either vintage or it's got to be young. I like vintage, kind of French lingerie with high-waists and corsets and stuff. And then, if you want to know what's cute, go and see what the girls are wearing in the Spearmint Rhino in Vegas. Girls need to look at what flatters them, rather than what might look good on somebody else. There is also something cute, for young girls, about cotton panties and simple stuff; not everything has to be a big production. I think girls have to go with their body type with all of the above. I like a girl who's got a commanding sexual presence, who can be dominating, who can wear… a girl who looks like my wife should wear a corset and fishnets and great shoes. I think a heavier girl trying to pull that off looks too forced. But I will say: ladies, rule number one is always have great shoes; rule number two is never take them off, no matter what.

HANDSOME DICK MANITOBA: I am a huge fan of what I call the pubescent stamp. The stamp was put in when I was 12/13 years old when I saw *Playboy* magazines. Actually one of my favourite sites online is the history of *Playboy* centrefolds. Not only because I can go look at Bebe Buell, who's a friend of mine, and a girl named Karen Hafter, from 1976 I think; she was in my home room in high school. Like any other memory recall – a smell, a song, a TV show – I can look at a *Playboy* centrefold and that brings me back to being 11 and 12 years old. And I think opening up those pages and seeing those naked girls had a profound effect on my life, so I tend to go back to those styles. I think they're deep in my psyche. Those styles of like negligees; girls with dark hair, puffed up with a white band around and white lipstick and those see-through, white, shorty negligees and everything's natural. Like that Sixties style and that type of underwear. See-through and sheer stuff tends to be my favourite. I'm not that into the super-thin anal floss underwear. I like more covering but showing; something that titillates and stirs the imagination more than overly obvious boobs plunging out.

JAMES KOTTAK: None! I think nothing trashy, just pasty, nice, soft pink, leopard underwear.

SEE-THROUGH AND SHEER STUFF TENDS TO BE MY FAVOURITE. I'M NOT THAT INTO THE SUPER-THIN ANAL FLOSS UNDERWEAR.

JESSE HUGHES: Hot lingerie, man? I've got so many favourites – my God! I like that sort of girl with the big bubble-butt and she's got a G-string poking up above the jeans, even though it's clichéd and lame, it's still horny. But then again, I like classic underwear. I like nice, thigh-high 'hose. I like knee-high socks with [Converse] All-Stars and that's it.

JIMMY ASHHURST: The French seem to have good ideas about lingerie. The French always seem to do it right… the French maid – all that sort of stuff – is quite invigorating.

JOEL O'KEEFFE: Well, when you're sitting in a restaurant and under the table your hand sneaks up her thigh, there's nothing more fun then finding she's got nothing on underneath! But if I had to pick, I'd say a white or black lace overlay stretch satin babydoll should do the trick.

LEMMY: Something called a teddy. You know those garments with a pair of knickers with it? I like the white ones. I'm a very virginal person – I'm not, but I like them to look like it.

NICKE BORG: I was talking to my tech today about the G-string. We were actually talking about the guitar G-string, which is the hardest one to tune – the hardest one to get in fucking control of – and I was thinking that there must be some kind of connection why they named the underwear G-strings, you know. So I would say a great ass with a hot little G-string.

ROB PATTERSON: I love fishnet stockings… ripped, of course.

TOBY RAND: A hot red G-string and a wifebeater – sexy as shit. Simple… and maybe a beanie as well. I love a beanie!

VAZQUEZ: Oh man, I love boy shorts. They're not thong panties but they kind of cover the ass, but not completely. It's in between a thong and granny panties. It looks fucking hot. It makes the ass cheeks look… it frames them so well.

Is there a method of removing clothing that turns you on most?

ACEY SLADE: With my eyes.

ADDE: Not really. Just rip them off.

ALLISON ROBERTSON: Not necessarily. I think that totally depends on the moment. I'm not really the kind of person who's into slowly taking clothes off. I never played strip poker but that's something that does not appeal to me; it sounds really boring. I'm more into like who cares, take it off, get it over with.

ANDREW W.K.: Depends what the clothing is. Perhaps the most sexy thing to me is a girl wearing a really tight, plain white T-shirt. Just a plain T-shirt, regular cotton or maybe a thinner cotton, with no bra. There's something about that, the way the fabric… that very soft, stretchy, jersey T-shirt fabric, even if it's one of those tank-tops or, as they call them, wifebeaters (although I never really liked that name for it). There's something about the way that fabric stretches and presses that things feel really good; the flesh feels really good through that fabric. And taking off that fabric, the way the bottom of the T-shirt as it's being lifted up over the body, the way it has to fight over the curves, the way it pulls against the plumper areas and then releases with hopefully a springy bounce. Taking off T-shirts is a real strong one; otherwise it's buttons, dresses and zippers. I like it when a woman removes her clothing. That's probably the most exciting.

BLASKO: I think slowly works out the best for me.

BRENT MUSCAT: If you can't wait and you're impatient, ripping stuff off is always fun.

BRUCE KULICK: That brings up the whole foreplay story and in some ways that's fun and in some ways just ripping the clothes off as quickly as you can and getting naked right away, getting into bed and jumping all over each other is the way to go. I do like the dance of having some clothes on, and then getting intimate and removing the clothes, rather than, 'OK, I'm naked in bed, now take me!' I think there is more fun in the undressing because let's face it, it's pretty obvious that you can be sexual if you're completely naked, but I think it's much harder when I grab my girlfriend and we just get to that hotel room and we're undressing as we're walking to the bed; we're kissing and grabbing each other. That's hot to me! By the time you wind up naked in bed you're just raring to go. But if it's like, 'OK, I'm taking a shower now and then I'm getting into bed,' well big deal! You probably go to bed naked anyway, so what's sexy about that? I'm not saying a naked girl isn't sexy, but it doesn't give that signal of, 'Hey, do you want me? Come get me.' That's why my girl knows to put on a nightie and she knows I'm going to respond to that.

CHIP Z'NUFF: Yes. Immediately, threads off. Immediately disrobing turns me on quickly.

COURTNEY TAYLOR-TAYLOR: The 14-year-old style, tight, confined space… kind of just hot and tugging. If the smart part of your brain finds it ridiculous but at the same time it's unstoppable, I like that. That's super fun and super sexy, super hot.

DANKO JONES: The whole removing clothes thing to me is kind of tedious. I like to walk into a room and it's already done and we're ready to go. I'm very impatient, let's put it that way.

DOUG ROBB: I guess slow is always the best way right? Teasing a little bit as you go. It depends on the mood: if the mood calls on the quick removal of clothing and that means ripping some of it in the process, then that's pretty fucking hot.

EVAN SEINFELD: If a girl's very attractive, I like to watch her undress herself slowly.

GINGER: Slowly, very slowly. There's no hurry is there? I do like to keep panties 'til last if it's a new girl, and shoes first to get her feeling comfortable and at home.

HANDSOME DICK MANITOBA: Yeah shredding it; ripping it off.

JAMES KOTTAK: No, just rip them off.

JESSE HUGHES: Absolutely, first you ply with alcohol… just joking. The key to removing clothing is a tricky one. You have to have the mood. I find that music is often an essential tool. For removing clothing, you need music that is slow and subtle because the serpent was the most subtle of all the creatures of the Garden and if you're going to defile the woman and beguile her, you've got to move in slow. Low lights are very helpful. Actually, I find it best to make it seem like, 'You can't take off my clothes,' you know what I mean? A little Br'er Rabbit with the girls never hurts. 'Please don't throw me in that briar patch.'

JIMMY ASHHURST: It depends on the circumstances. I believe there are certain times when it should be as quickly as possible, and there are other times where you want to prolong the excitement as best you can. Sometimes, leaving it all on for quite some time is a good move.

JOEL O'KEEFFE: Smooth and slow or rough and fast, or both, get the same result.

LEMMY: No, any way will do as long as it goes.

NICKE BORG: It depends on how much clothing they wear. When you live here in Sweden, you have to have that in mind because they usually have a lot of clothes on in the first place 'cause it's fucking cold. I think you should keep most of your stuff on as long as possible – that's a turn-on I think – and then let your partner remove them in a very sexual way. I usually go to a lot of strip clubs everywhere and you can tell if that city is really cool or not by the way the girls remove their clothing.

ROB PATTERSON: The fastest?

TOBY RAND: If the girl removes your clothing first – your top half – and she does a striptease for you really fuckin' slowly, so you don't know what she's going to do next.

VAZQUEZ: As long as the light is on and I get to see everything that's happening then I'm more than happy to be there. It doesn't have to be a striptease, you know?

How much should someone show or hide with their choice of clothing?

ACEY SLADE: If a girl's showing too much and is too aggressive, I'm probably thinking I'm just someone else in line, but that's OK sometimes. I remember reading about a Seventies rock drummer who would bring these school teachers on the bus and just wreck them.

BLASKO: I think that's up to the individual. Like, I'm not into the baggy style of clothes that makes someone look fat or whatever, but there's a fine line. You can rock some cleavage and show a little ass crack every now and then as long as it's somehow done in a non-slutty way. There are different ways that can be done, but there are fine lines. I think it's up to the individual as to where you'd see something like that.

COURTNEY TAYLOR-TAYLOR: As much as possible – show the silhouette but hide 69% of the texture. I like arms and shoulders exposed, but other than that I think a pair of tight, faded 1971-era bell bottoms with cowboy boots and a little worn-out T-shirt is just the best; there's nothing like it.

NICKE BORG: There's something really sexy about a girl who dresses really well and you don't have to see her naked, but it's also sexy to have a naked body with very little clothes on.

ROB PATTERSON: If you have good style that doesn't matter.

TOBY RAND: I love a chick who would wear a rock T-shirt – and not the dresses with the fancy glitter and all that stuff – a chick with some fuckin' hot tight jeans, with maybe her ass crack showing just a touch, no bra and a tight T-shirt… and a beanie.

VAZQUEZ: I think show as much as you've got. Like David Lee Roth once said, 'You'd better use it up before it gets old.'

COPULATION

"OVER IN THE FAR EAST
THEY'RE A LITTLE BIT
DIFFERENT. THEY LIKE
THE BACK DOOR"

What position always makes your partner go crazy?

ACEY SLADE: Probably when I'm between their legs.

ADDE: I have to say the missionary because it's so personal. I need to have sex with somebody who looks me in the eyes. It's really, really hard to be with somebody who's shy and stuff like that, and they don't look you in the eyes; I don't get that connection. Missionary gives me that.

ALLISON ROBERTSON: I don't know; I've had a couple of different partners and they're all different. I think for the most part, I think with most guys the more they can see the better. So I think guys like when they can see you and your face. But I don't really know; to me they're all good.

ANDREW W.K.: It seems like the reverse. I don't really like the word doggy-style but that's the way most people refer to it. From behind, every time, with every girl.

BLASKO: I think doggy-style is the answer to this one.

BRENT MUSCAT: The reverse cowgirl is pretty fun. I like doggy-style, when you can reach around and rub the girl on the front; that's always pretty good. So I would say… I don't know what you would call it, but it's almost like doggy-style where the girl is laying on her side but you can reach around and play with their clitoris. I think that's a good one for the girls.

> I LIKE DOGGY-STYLE, WHEN YOU CAN REACH AROUND AND RUB THE GIRL ON THE FRONT; THAT'S ALWAYS PRETTY GOOD.

BRUCE KULICK: I think I'm a good lover and I've been told that. And oddly enough, on top, I seem to do it interestingly enough, even though that's the most boring in some ways. I do like when a girl's on top because you get to see them in their glory, which is fun. I'm very tall and I've dated all different shapes, I have to admit. My current girl is a little taller than petite, but depending on your partner's shape, some positions just don't work: one being doggy-style. That's great with some bodies and with some the angle's not right and it just ain't going to work. That's a dance that you have to make sure that you and your partner fit. I'm up for all of them; I enjoy them all, but ultimately I'm only going to enjoy the ones that make sense with the physique of my lover and that's what's going to make it work. I seem to enjoy them all, but I won't do them with a girl that it just doesn't work for, or they don't like that. I find a lot of girls really like if the guy can be on top. They feel dominated and most of them, if they are going to have an orgasm they probably will, especially if they're really turned on of course.

CHIP Z'NUFF: Sixty-ten, which is a sixty-nine but one more.

DANKO JONES: Doggy-style or missionary. Standing up has always been a turn-on for them, but to be honest, I get tired.

DOUG ROBB: My wife loves being on top. I think she puts her legs back straight but kind of sitting on top of me. It works every time.

EVAN SEINFELD: Women seem to love doggy-style, no two ways about it. I've interviewed hundreds of women on camera for rockstarpimp.com and very unanimously, I'd say 85% of all women prefer doggy-style to any other position. Kind of like, they become really firm with their knees under themselves. I do often hurt girls in that position. I kind of like that and I think they kind of like that too. Finding that point between pain and pleasure… I think women like to feel overwhelmed. And my personal favourite is definitely missionary. Me, I like to see the look on their face when I've got my whole dick inside them.

HANDSOME DICK MANITOBA: I don't want to cop out but nine years later we're still pretty excited by regular stuff. We're really not kinky. We don't need like six extra people or chandeliers. The regular stuff is still absolutely thrilling.

JESSE HUGHES: The position where I am exactly right up inside of them… just kidding. Some girls are different, man. The most amazing sex I've ever had with my girl was on all-fours I think. Actually, all-fours, head down. All-fours on the bed – that's it!

JIMMY ASHHURST: The ones where they're on top: at this stage in the game, the more work they can do, the better off I am.

JOEL O'KEEFFE: Her body is a temple and her pussy is the front door, so make sure you make a big entrance and she'll want you coming back for more.

LEMMY: Probably standing outside the house shouting through the window. I don't know; let me think. It's difficult to describe really, but I know what it is.

NICKE BORG: From behind I think, or like, half behind. There's something with that fucking doggy-style. Usually I don't give any thoughts about that, but even the kinkiest girls tend to think there's something about having sex doggy-style.

TOBY RAND: I think it's called the reverse cowboy; that always works. It's when you are either lying or just sitting down, maybe on the edge of the bed, and the girl's faced the other way and you're both looking in a mirror at each other as you do it. That's always pretty hot. I find that visual is always a good way.

VAZQUEZ: Always from behind! Women fucking love that. You know what man? I don't have a huge dick, so if I'm behind them, they're getting bang for their buck. So long as I'm not standing on the bed, I'm cool with that – I can keep going as long as I want.

Have you found people from different countries prefer certain positions?

ACEY SLADE: I don't know about positions, but there are differences. European girls are definitely freer and easier. Japanese girls make the weirdest noises, which can actually come in really handy because I used to date a girl who would make really, really strange noises and it would just make me last for a really long time. The longer I lasted, the weirder the noises would go and I was so glad we didn't have the lights on because I was just in tears laughing at these strange noises. So yeah, Japanese girls definitely make weird noises, but as far as positions I haven't noticed anything.

ADDE: No, not really, but I used to live in Los Angeles and I used to date this black girl and she was really, really good at sucking cock and she told me after that she'd been listening to N.W.A. her whole life and they have a song about how to suck dick and she was really, really good. It was like… amazing!

ALLISON ROBERTSON: No! I'm a pretty good girl. I haven't done like every guy in every town and every city, but I definitely think that most guys are pretty boring. By what they pretend they do, I think a lot of them just like being on top, and I'm including people from other countries.

ANDREW W.K.: I've never been with a girl who has not lived the majority of her life in the United States. You're the first person to ask. I've never even realised that before. One of the girls lived a long time in Canada, so I guess that kind of counts, but hardly counts because it's so like America. That's a great question and in some ways I would like to have had more research in that area. I put my sexual energy into more long-term relationships.

BLASKO: I wouldn't really be a good gauge on that. I just haven't been through many different countries.

BRENT MUSCAT: The girls in England are always really fun and pretty wild from my experience. Japanese girls are always very fun too. In Japan, something about sex seems more natural to them and they're not super hung-up about sex. In America, from the way America was formed on sort of Christian values, there are a lot of people kind of hung-up about sex. Not everyone; it's opened up a lot but there's still… The way America was formed was like Protestant or something, where virginity was a virtue and you shouldn't have pre-marital sex and you should only do the missionary position. There are some people who are a little hung-up about all that, so a country like Japan has a totally different culture and there are not a whole lot of hang-ups about it.

BRUCE KULICK: I can't really say that; it's interesting. I have been fortunate enough to say I have dated some women around the world and I can't tell you that, 'Oh, wow! Over here they like it this way.' I think with sex it's universal. I do know certain cultures get a little more… you know, the South Americans are very butt orientated (and I'm not saying that as an anal sex thing). So does that mean they like it more doggy-style? I don't know. The girls that I like down there, we seemed to have sex just the way that I would with a girl from New York City or LA. You'll hear certain things; supposedly there are certain connections with certain cultures, but I haven't really experienced anything radically weird about that in any way – geographic specific. Good sex is good sex and it doesn't matter where it comes from.

CHIP Z'NUFF: I've toured the world but I haven't boned in every single city that's for sure. I want to be safe out there. I'm in a tough business and you can't trust everybody. With that being said, it's different everywhere. Japan's very strange, I know that. Over in the Far East they're a little bit different. They like the back door. Everywhere is different of course, but we carry ourselves a certain way and the apple doesn't fall far from the tree. I don't think you stray too far away when you're in a different country. There's different cultures and there's different people but you still are what you are.

COURTNEY TAYLOR-TAYLOR: Closer to the equator is definitely dirtier and more ass orientated, and I think they tend to get more oral as you head to the poles.

DANKO JONES: No. I haven't really observed that, in terms of geography, no.

DOUG ROBB: No, and the only reason I can say that is that I've never had sex with somebody outside of this country [USA].

EVAN SEINFELD: I've had sex in probably a hundred countries around the world and I think people are people. I think girls like to get fucked from behind and from the front, and I think girls will get on top wherever you give them a chance. I think the most uptight girls are in England. I think England probably has the least attractive girls. I think the position that I least like is a British girl naked and talking. It seems popular in Britain for them to want to talk while they're naked.

JAMES KOTTAK: I've never really noticed a correlation with that. That's for sure; not at all.

JESSE HUGHES: I find that different countries allow for the sexual scenarios to be under certain terms, which requires it to be fast, furious and over with. Some cultures somehow devalue women in a way that makes them seem almost inconsequential, so I'm sure that sex is probably like getting fondled by your gym teacher. The country definitely dictates the position. America seems to want to be like the kings of the world, so we like a lot of positions.

JIMMY ASHHURST: Most of the experiences I've had outside of this country, the positions have normally been out in the alley by the dumpster and things of that nature. It hadn't really occurred to me man; I'll have to look into that. In Japan there's a cultural difference there that I'm not quite hip to. I always end up traumatised when I'm there because it's like the language barrier, etc, so you never quite know what's going on… and I think they like it that way. It's like, 'Is she enjoying this, or is she going to call the cops, or what?' It's a bit of a mystery – the mysterious Orient.

LEMMY: No, no I haven't really. I think everybody's more or less the same. As long as it feels good, we do it, right?

NICKE BORG: No, not really actually.

TOBY RAND: Yes, South American women love to be really expressive with their body movement and they want to be seen and they want to show, so they love to be on top.

VAZQUEZ: No, it's all very universal from what I've experienced.

Any good ways to encourage a partner to try a new position?

ACEY SLADE: I'm open to anything. It's pretty cool if a girl takes the reins. It can be a little awkward at first sometimes. All of a sudden you've got an appendage in someone's face that wasn't intended to be there, so you're like, 'OK, stick with me. We're not staying in this position; we're going to go to the starboard bow area.'

CHIP Z'NUFF: Be nice, trustworthy and gentle. Usually a little alcohol or drugs will help bamboozle that person into trying anything.

COURTNEY TAYLOR-TAYLOR: We don't really sit around and plan it out. Wherever you are, that's the position.

JOEL O'KEEFFE: Pick 'em up and put 'em where you want 'em – no questions asked.

TOBY RAND: I think the best way is to just do; to ease your way to do it. Or make it a bit of fun; make it into a game like, 'I dare you, if you dare me' kind of thing. I like to make it fun and actually laugh and play during sex. Make everyone feel comfortable – it's important.

VAZQUEZ: Hell dude, I'm an entertainer so I do what I want. So it's just like, 'OK, I promise you you'll like it.'

What's the strangest position a partner has encouraged you to try?

ACEY SLADE: Probably with her doing a handstand against the wall.

ADDE: Probably me being positioned like a girl. Like, I'm riding the girl like the girl with my cock. That felt kind of awkward.

ALLISON ROBERTSON: To be honest, I don't think I've gotten lucky enough for anybody to have ever done that. I'm usually more adventurous, like more into trying things and usually the guys I'm with are more like, 'Oh that hurts' or 'I'm uncomfortable with that'. I've dated a lot of babies in my life; I'll be honest. So I actually don't have the privilege to say something wild for that question.

ANDREW W.K.: I did have the very good fortune of being with a girl who worked as a stripper for quite some time. Actually, I don't really know how long she had been doing it, but it seemed like she had been doing it for a while. She was young though, so it couldn't have been that long. She was staying at my house and we were having intimate relations and she was very open-minded and very advanced in the way of sex, in terms of concept. Now, I don't remember enough really if the sex was very good, but she was the one who wanted to do stuff to me. So that by far was the weirdest, meaning she put her fingers inside me, she wanted to use a vibrator on me, to which I said no – we were going to work our way up to that. I was really pushing myself into a realm I had never gone and I was only able to do it because I had a few friends who had explained that they had done that before with girls. They didn't really like it but it was one of those experiences in life that they felt great for having tried. I guess I tried it and having her be the dominant force was a weird feeling. We did it one time I think. It was definitely introducing me to a part of my body that I had never really interacted with before. That was really life-changing, just to have had done it. It was pretty interesting, but I never went there with any other girl. I never felt the urge to after that. It's interesting because it wasn't the best sex at all; it was the most crazy in concept.

BLASKO: As long as there's intercourse involved, I don't know that it's ever all that terribly strange. Like, 'Can I put a dildo on and fuck you in the ass?' is kind of where I draw the line.

BRENT MUSCAT: Hmm, well I think I've tried all the different positions. I don't think there was anything *that* strange. Doing it in the front seat of a car you have to get in some awkward positions in order to do it. I think I've tried everything so I don't know if there are any strange positions; I think I've tried all the possible positions.

BRUCE KULICK: Oh that's a tough question and I'm not sure I can remember anything where it was that unusual. I don't pick very domineering girls because that doesn't do it for me. So if I'm kind of leading the dance, shall I say, we're probably going to be in positions that I'm kind of used to. I'm not that kind of person who's like, 'Let's do it standing. OK, I'm putting you on the table now.' So I don't have anything really interesting to answer that one with.

CHIP Z'NUFF: Head-first down a bidet. In Japan, I hear that head-first down a bidet is interesting. In a bathtub of ice cubes. None of these I tried by the way. Those are two that come to mind right away.

DANKO JONES: Nothing really crazy for me. Not in my experiences; nothing outrageous, like from a chandelier or anything, nothing like that for me. I've done some crazy things, but nothing in terms of position-wise.

DOUG ROBB: You could consider me fortunate or unfortunate, but I've never had any request where I've been like, 'Are you fucking kidding me? Really?' So, nothing I haven't seen in any strong adult movie or rated-R movie; it's pretty standard.

EVAN SEINFELD: I've had a lot of girls want to get really elaborate into like a play-rape, play-home invasion kind of thing, where they want me to like… They get real specific, like, 'I want you to crawl in my window and wear a black ski mask and then I want you to take me and tie me up and hide me in a closet and then fuck me against my will.' And I'm like, 'Well if you ask me to do it, it's not really against your will then is it?' I've had lots of girls that wanted to fuck in public. I've had pretty serious requests where other women want me to fuck them in front of their boyfriends or something. I've certainly had my share of girls who want me to kind of dominate them; that's a really common request.

HANDSOME DICK MANITOBA: If it's not in my repertoire, at this stage in my life I'm not planning on getting experimental. You never know what's around the corner but I guess I'm kind of bland sexually in terms of tits and ass and vagina. All the basic stuff is still absolutely enough for me. It's still a great enough invention, there's nothing boring about it and I don't think it needs to be added to.

GINGER: In the middle of the road in traffic rush hour.

JESSE HUGHES: You know that Karma Sutra shit, all that hippie shit? Girls get all wrapped up in that and that's cool and stuff to look at the ancient porno and all that jazz, but this girl tried to get me in a position where she wanted me to spread my legs somehow. I'm not totally against that but I'm a cowboy, you know what I'm saying?

JIMMY ASHHURST: Duct-taped to the wall always sticks out in my memory. Duct tape – it's fucking amazing stuff really… and it's in every road case. You can actually really support a human being. This was put to the test and I proved it. Next time I see you, we'll try and find a willing participant and I'll show you; you can actually duct tape one to the wall.

I'VE HAD PRETTY SERIOUS REQUESTS WHERE OTHER WOMEN WANT ME TO FUCK THEM IN FRONT OF THEIR BOYFRIENDS OR SOMETHING

LEMMY: I don't think anyone has encouraged me to try a strange one. Isn't that weird? You'd think they would have with all my years in rock'n'roll. I don't think there's anything that's really surprised me, but I'm pretty hard to surprise.

NICKE BORG: Being tied up on a big cross, and she asked me if it is OK if she wears a gas mask, so I was like, 'OK' This was at a strip bar.

ROB PATTERSON: Umm… I could answer that, but my friends would make fun of me.

TOBY RAND: The strangest was to be like a scissor. I'd have my legs open and she'd have her legs open but one of my legs would be under her and the other on top, and I'd have to pull her with my hands and kind of do a scissor-thing at the same time. It was really interesting.

VAZQUEZ: Honestly, I don't think anybody's ever asked me to do anything really fucked up or anything. Sex is real simple man: it's four-on-the-floor man. It's all you need.

DARING LOCATIONS

"MY WIFE AND I ARE CERTAINLY EXHIBITIONISTS. WE'VE HAD SEX UP IN THE EIFFEL TOWER"

What's the craziest place you've had sex in?

ACEY SLADE: A cemetery in Japan. It was really funny because this girl didn't speak English so well and I had mapped it out on the way to the hotel beforehand. It was like dawn the next morning and the girl and I were in the room, and I'm like, 'Let's go for a walk' and her English was terrible and my Japanese wasn't much better. We were kind of in the middle of things and she was like, 'Where are you taking me? What is going on here?' So we went to the cemetery.

ADDE: Probably when I lived in Hollywood: I had sex on the rooftop of the building where I lived and there was like the chimney. I put her on it and we had sex, but it made so much noise that my neighbour came up and was like, 'What the fuck is going on on the roof?' because we were lying right above his stove and he could hear the sound... like big birds or something – humping.

ALLISON ROBERTSON: Probably... well, I don't think it's crazy but there's the [tour] bus and every band does that. So probably it's kind of normal, but it also feels crazy when for instance the doors don't lock or the bunk is really uncomfortable because it's like having sex in a coffin or something. Also, I guess maybe like a moving car could be something that's kind of dangerous. It's hard to say because it all depends on how you look at it, but they're all pretty generic things if you're in a band.

ANDREW W.K.: I don't think that there's been any locations I would consider crazy. I guess it felt pretty crazy to me to have sexual relations in the tour bus in my bunk because it was so close to other people. For me, right there is the craziest thing I've ever done. To hear other people's voices in the other rooms, to be like there was someone two feet away from you in pretty much every direction when you're in your bunk on the bus. Plus you're so cramped in the bunk; it's a very small space to work within. In terms of a public place, I guess I've done a few things in a car but I don't think I've ever done anything like that. That never appealed to me for some reason; I don't know why.

BLASKO: This is probably going to come off tame in comparison to the other dudes you've talked to, but for me maybe like the rooftop of a hotel or like in the bathroom at a club. I'm sure that's pretty standard shit but to me that's about as crazy as I've ever got.

BRENT MUSCAT: I got a blowjob inside a dark corner of a club before. Of course the back seat of my car. At school, when I was in high school with some girl in like the back room of a classroom. When I was a teenager with one of my teenage girlfriends in the front living room of her house looking out the window making sure her parents weren't coming home – that was pretty crazy.

BRUCE KULICK: I did have a slightly aggressive girlfriend for a while; she was just raring to go any time. I was touring at the time and she'd be very happy to do it in the car. Sometimes that's fine for me but it's not if I don't feel like I'm private, where I'm like, 'Well the tour bus is only 50 yards away.' So I'd be like, 'I think I'm into this; no, I'm not into it.' I know that's a turn-on for some people – the public sexual thing – and I remember when I was really young and first getting excited with girls and going to the park because I was living at my parents' and everything. I was horny enough that I could be in the park in New York by the World's Fair where the big Unisphere is from the *Men in Black* movie; that's where I used to go. I remember one time doing it there! I mean, that's ridiculous to think of now. I remember one time going at it with one of my first girlfriends and a cop drove by and shone the light and I was like 'Urghh', but he just wanted to be sure I wasn't raping someone. We both looked at the cop with that same look of, 'Please don't bust us, we're really having a good time', so he carried on and said like, 'Don't worry about it.' But that's what he was looking for; he wasn't looking to tell me not to do that. He just thinks, 'Is the girl going to scream?' Obviously if I was raping her, the girl would be screaming and I'd be totally busted but no, we were totally having a great time. But that's something you do when you're 18 and you don't do later in life. The public thing just never really appealed to me. I guess I'm just a little more reserved than that, that's all.

CHIP Z'NUFF: Roppongi, Japan and a little club called The Lexington Queen. I was hanging out there and Julian Lennon came in with Lucy, this chick from Robert Plant's band. We all hung out and cocktailed and had a great time. Afterwards, Julian asked if my brother and I would like to join him for a late-night dinner, which would be four in the morning, OK? So we hit up some Mexican restaurant – great food, great time. I'm really not a big drinker but I was cocktailing there just to keep up with him and I ran into two goddesses out there (both Japanese girls) and they took me back to the Roppongi Prince Hotel where we were staying. That was very interesting! They insisted on having the lights off. I was concerned because I wasn't sure if anything was tucked and perhaps there was some camera for a TV show. The last thing I wanted was to be caught in the act where I can't bamboozle my way out of it. However, they tempted me and they won and it was a good experience. I woke up in the morning though and the bed was completely full of blood. For one of the girls it was that time of the month and I couldn't tell because the lights were off. It was a really good time until that. She was very embarrassed. I remember I told her, 'Don't worry about it' and I tore the sheets off and put them away and threw them out of the room and tried to make her feel better, but the damage was already done.

COURTNEY TAYLOR-TAYLOR: The dark room at college, but nothing crazy.

DANKO JONES: It's pretty common but an alley. It was more of a garage; someone's garage was open and we went in. We were walking on a residential street, someone's garage was open and we just went in and did it.

DOUG ROBB: Some people get turned-on by having sex in public or in a place where they might get caught but that doesn't necessarily heighten anything for me. I have done some very sexual things on a plane; not necessarily having sex but pretty much everything else you can do – and that's not in the bathroom; that's just in the seat.

EVAN SEINFELD: My wife and I are certainly exhibitionists. We've had sex up in the Eiffel Tower; in dozens of different airplanes. There's something really hot about having sex on an aeroplane with your partner, but there's something really over the edge about having sex with a stranger on an aeroplane. I think that's really daring to have never seen the person [before].

THERE'S SOMETHING REALLY HOT ABOUT HAVING SEX ON AN AEROPLANE WITH YOUR PARTNER, BUT THERE'S SOMETHING REALLY OVER THE EDGE ABOUT HAVING SEX WITH A STRANGER ON AN AEROPLANE.

HANDSOME DICK MANITOBA: I go back to the Seventies with this: the first two sexual experiences in my life were outdoors. There was a point in my life where my nickname was Nature Boy Manitoba. I think I should change back to that from Handsome Dick because there are just too many dick jokes with Handsome Dick. It gets a bit much after 35 years. No one gets it; it's a professional wrestling name, but I should go back to this name if I could – Nature Boy Manitoba – nobody tortures you with it. Anyway, I got that name because there was an endless list of outdoor sexual activity. The first one was when I was about 15/16 years old and about 50 feet behind this bench where all the kids used to hang out at this park in the Bronx. I remember this girl was masturbating me and when I came, people turned around and started clapping. And like a week later I had sex with the girl. In those days it was like the dawn of Quaaludes and I was always buzzed on Quaaludes, which is like a dry drunk, mellow feeling. It's a muscle relaxant, so I was always kind of out of it. I had sex with a girl on the New York State throughway. I had sex with a girl in a park in St Louis when I was working as a bartender there for two weeks in 1983 I believe… that sort of thing.

JAMES KOTTAK: The ladies bathroom at Harrah's Casino in Laughlin, Nevada. We got thrown out and yes, that was with Athena. Athena and I have been thrown out of every casino in Laughlin. There's about 14 of them and we've been thrown out of every single one of them at one time or another.

JESSE HUGHES: In rock'n'roll, you're provided with opportunity sometimes and a variety of crazy scenarios. Behind a church I've had sex. I've had sex in a Greyhound bus before in Indio, California. Let's see, where else have I had sex? Oh God, OK I've got to tell you this I guess: at a Parent Teacher Association meeting at the McCallum Theatre for a fundraiser. I had sex with one of the teacher's wives in one of the dust closets.

JIMMY ASHHURST: Japan!

LEMMY: I had sex on top of one of those photo booths in Chester Station once during rush hour and nobody looked up. People don't look up you know; it's funny. Also the Roundhouse in London; outside the restaurant part of it there was a cart with shafts – you know one of those old carts with the big wheels – and I fucked a chick in there once and her legs were hanging over the sides and she was going 'Ow, ow, ow' and nobody looked up again; it's funny. Where else? Oh, all kinds of places. On a tube train. This chick got on it about six in the morning after doing an all-nighter and we got into the last carriage on the train and the cab was open (they have a cab at both ends) and we got in there. She was going down on me standing up in the cab and we're pulling into the station and dropping people off and I'm waving to them, with a blonde head bopping about on me. The most outrageous was probably when a chick jumped up onstage and blew me while we were playing, early on in Motörhead's career.

NICKE BORG: Usually I'm not too much of a wilderness guy – too many ants in your pants. I've never really fucked in an airplane either, which most people think that since you're in a band you've joined that 10,000 Miles Club or whatever. I did not, but I did get a hand job once – but that was on a train, so I don't have much to brag about. So, craziest place? I don't know.

ROB PATTERSON: In a movie theatre when I was 17, in the row right behind my girlfriend's mother.

VAZQUEZ: I had a girlfriend and she was working in a dry cleaners and it was kind of a populated area where it was. The front counter was literally like six feet from the door and there was some sort of religious place next door – it was like a strip mall. I just got behind the counter and pulled down her pants and went at it. It was great 'cause people were like walking by as we were doing it and they had no idea what was going on. It was fantastic man – God bless that girl!

What's the best way to avoid getting caught in the act?

ACEY SLADE: Being quiet. But then again, I think getting caught is kind of the fun part.

ADDE: I don't know any best ways – if you get caught, you get caught.

ANDREW W.K.: Being very, very quiet. I like being very quiet anyway. I always thought that was pretty cool. I've had girls that are more vocal and that can be great, but I also like girls when they've been very quiet because you end up hearing other things. When you're not screaming or vocalising, there's endless sounds in a way to focus in on. Being quiet was always a good thing, whether you were at your parents' house, your friend's house or wherever you are. I thought it was respectful too. I've had people where I swear they've been trying to be really loud so other people would hear them and that would be a turn-on for them. I thought that was really inconsiderate. Clearly they were getting off on that idea, but I found it very invasive and very aggressive in sort of a disturbing way.

BLASKO: I think that if you're out in public or whatever, the danger element part of it is to potentially be caught, which is the excitement factor. So I don't know that you're really going to try to ensure that you don't get caught.

CHIP Z'NUFF: Don't do it. Simple. There's always repercussions later, no matter what it is. Just be able to say no. It's tough, but you'll feel better about it the next day. Take care of yourself.

DANKO JONES: I guess you'd do it in a dark alley at night. That's what I did.

DOUG ROBB: On a plane have some blankets to cover you and make sure it's one of those night flights. The best way not to get caught is to do it in a place where you're not going to get caught! Just have it thought out. Spontaneous sex is the kind of sex you might get caught out doing.

EVAN SEINFELD: I think having sex in public is like writing graffiti: you have to just do it. If you're really looking around and worrying about it you draw attention to yourself and will get caught. Just stay cool and stay in the moment, and try to just blend in with your surroundings. I remember me and Tera on one of our first dates had sex at the Long Beach Airport in like a crowded parking garage. And like, not in the car, leaning over the back of it. We had planes and helicopters going overhead; we were both so turned on. Tera and I love to have sex in like department store dressing rooms where there are obviously cameras.

We want to imagine some guy like beating off on the other side going, 'Oh my God! I can't believe this.'

GINGER: What's wrong with getting caught in the act? Sometimes the thrill of being caught can heighten the sexual experience to incredible levels.

HANDSOME DICK MANITOBA: The only fear I have of getting caught in the act is by my son. I don't want my son to have that one traumatic moment that defines his sexual life because he's like, 'Oh my God! I opened up the door and there they were!' That's a great fear of mine. But with the other kind of getting caught in the act, I was always a one-girl-at-a-time kind of guy. I'm not that good at being heinous and hiding stuff; it's too nerve-racking.

JAMES KOTTAK: Do it at home in the bathroom with the door locked.

JESSE HUGHES: You never hide anything by intention; you simply leave it out in the open. It is what it is. The only people getting spotted by cops while smoking a joint are the dudes looking back and forth like they're at a fucking tennis match.

JIMMY ASHHURST: Always try and find a door with a lock on it. If that's not possible, which it often isn't, you have to have a good buddy and you have to appoint that person as the lookout.

JOEL O'KEEFFE: Well it really depends on how well you adapt to your surroundings. Like, if you're in the park, the rotunda or a thick spot of bushes will work. If it's in an elevator, hit the emergency stop button. If it's in the cinema, up the back or in the restroom as not too many people go there when the movie is on. The best time in the restroom on a plane is when they turn the cabin lights out because everyone goes to sleep, or if it's at the beach, do it vertical in the water as any onlookers will just think you're very happy to see each other.

LEMMY: Go to another country. Do it in a bank vault.

ROB PATTERSON: Don't get caught!

VAZQUEZ: I don't even worry about it. Once I'm in the zone and once I'm thinking about it, I could be in a room full of people having sex and I don't fucking care.

Any good locations you recommend to try at least once in your lifetime?

ACEY SLADE: One time in Central Park, New York City, and one time on the beach on the Gold Coast, Australia.

ALLISON ROBERTSON: Well I think it would be nice to do it on a beach. To me that's the ultimate. There are people around and to me the beach is really sexy, so I think everybody should try the beach.

BLASKO: I've always been curious about the Mile-High Club. I've never done it but it seems like the element of danger might be cool, so I'm going to recommend that one, even though I've never done it – I'll recommend it for myself.

BRENT MUSCAT: The beach is good. I think a car is a must; the back seat of a car is always fun. A tour bus is good too; the back lounge of the tour bus is pretty fun.

BRUCE KULICK: Well I do think that the back of a tour bus is fun. Not exactly public, but it certainly isn't in your hotel room or your home. I could imagine a beach being really sexy, even though I hate sand so I wouldn't even go there on a beach. To be honest, that park experience was a lot of fun; nothing wrong with a lot of grass and a real breeze on a nice summer night in New York.

CHIP Z'NUFF: Amsterdam, absolutely! There's something in the water out there: you can hold a rig [erection] for hours and hours out there. I don't know what it is. It's something in the food, maybe it's in the water; it's something out there. Plus you're around all this smoke and everything's free. There are no hassles or anything. Another good place to go to I would recommend is Australia if you're an American. They seem to be very fond of us. Last but not least, Poland. Poland is really good, absolutely. They're wide open, they treat their men terrific, they're classy, they're clean, articulate, and all they care about is having a great time and they're not about smothering.

COURTNEY TAYLOR-TAYLOR: When you're all still living at your parents' house, try your friend's parents' walk-in closet at a party at their house when they're gone. That is one of the most amazing young sexual experiences.

DANKO JONES: No, just to get some is good enough – wherever you can get it. That's what I have to say.

DOUG ROBB: The beach. Not that I thought it was so amazing, but I just remembered that I had sex on the beach.

EVAN SEINFELD: I think everybody should certainly try a really public place, like a shopping mall or a football field, to see if it turns them on, because I think you either like it or you don't. I'm a fan. There are lots of things with people that turn them on that don't interest me, but definitely having sex outside in public... I think it's about the spontaneity though. Like, for all you know I'm getting a blowjob right now as we speak.

HANDSOME DICK MANITOBA: Oh, you've got to do the beach! Anything where the environment adds detail, like there's wind. Also the thing about outdoors and the beach is there's danger. I mean, you don't want to do danger where some knuckleheads are going to come up or you're going to get arrested, but the air of danger, the possibility of danger rather than a locked, closed door. The wind and the smells and the unknown, that's what I recommend you have to do at least once.

JAMES KOTTAK: Oh of course, down on the beach. Or just after a party and you're out in the car and you pull off on to the side of the road; that works.

JESSE HUGHES: In the trunk of a killer's car.

JIMMY ASHHURST: If you haven't done it in the back of a tour bus, I suggest everyone should have that opportunity. I encourage all the women who read this that haven't yet to give us a jingle next time we're around.

JOEL O'KEEFFE: I know it's a cliché but there's no better way to make a long haul flight exciting than getting it on in the restroom.

LEMMY: Up a tree. In a wishing well. In a bar, at the bar. I once got blown at the bar in New York City I remember.

NICKE BORG: On a mountain top somewhere... on skis.

ROB PATTERSON: On top of a car.

VAZQUEZ: I would have to say outside – not outside at night, but outside during the day. There's just something real special about the sunshine hitting your balls while you're fucking. I don't know how to describe it. I would say avoid the beach because of the sand factor, so do it in your backyard.

DATING & COURTSHIP

"THE GIRL WILL LET YOU KNOW. GIRLS ARE IN CHARGE OF RELATIONSHIPS; SHE'LL TELL YOU"

What raunchy pick-up line always works with you?

ACEY SLADE: I don't really have a raunchy one but mine's usually, 'Do you want to go to the bus and watch a movie?' It's terrible because I'm not on tour right now and I'm single, so I don't know what to say. I'm lost. I need to go to that Anthony Robbins guy's school to see how to pick-up girls because I have no idea.

ADDE: I'm not the type of guy that uses them. I just want to be down-to-earth; a gentleman. I don't have a standard phrase.

ALLISON ROBERTSON: No, I hate pick-up lines and I usually don't like guys at all that come after me unless they've got really good lines. I have to say that I like it when a guy just isn't mean for one thing because I seem to attract guys who go, 'Hey, your solo sucked' or whatever. I attract that kind of hair-pulling thing from some guys where they make fun of you and they think it's going to make you feel like, 'Oh, I want to have sex with that guy.' I'm much more interested if somebody's just nice and treats me like they respect me. They follow what I do on stage but they don't treat me like I think I'm any better than they are, because I really don't like when people treat me like I'm different from other people. Just because you play guitar doesn't mean you're really manly. Just because you're in a band doesn't mean you're a slut or whatever. So I just like it when someone comes up to me and says, 'Hey, that's cool what you do and I do this.' To me it's much more sexy when they're confident and don't try out all these stupid lines, or ass-kissing.

ANDREW W.K.: I got really into being very direct so I'd say, 'Would you like to kiss and make out?' That usually worked, but I never tried it on someone by just walking up to them out of the blue. I don't know if that counts as a pick-up line; maybe that's a proposition line. I learned from these older guys around me who would always walk up and say, 'Hi, my name is Andrew' (or whatever their name was) and that worked very well because I don't think any girl ever didn't at least say hi back. So that got them talking and then once you got their name, you could use their name as a way to start with and you could tell from their voice if you've never heard them speak before, like do they have an accent? Things can really open up. It seems so simple and silly, but it gives the girl your name, how you say your name, how you carry yourself. Introducing yourself is a very standard way of breaking the ice but there's a reason it's used so often. But it seems like with women and your typical pick-up line, sometimes you walk up and don't say your name first; you'd say a line first about how she looks or, 'Can I buy you a drink?', etc. Saying your name first is also putting yourself out there first, being vulnerable first and laying yourself down on the line first. It helps create a better dynamic.

BLASKO: I always thought lines were kind of cheesy. I don't know that people ever try to use lines on me.

BRENT MUSCAT: I've never really used pick-up lines. If I did, it just kind of comes out naturally; you say stupid stuff and kind of joke. The main thing is to be friends with someone first and just talk normally about things you have in common. I'm not a fan of pick-up lines. I think the best thing is to just be yourself and be natural.

BRUCE KULICK: Oh boy! Here's another thing: I've found that some of the girls who have been attracted to me is because I say things off the cuff. I don't have a pick-up line. I'll tell you the line that turned on my girl – the one I'm dating now – and I didn't even plan it. It wasn't really told towards her but it was something I said in front of her that turned her on enough to make her know. I was checking out my guitars (I have various different backline trucks for the Grand Funk shows that I do) and I hadn't seen these guitars in probably a month or two, so I was just looking at them. She's into music and she was going to be introducing me for the show as she works for the local radio station on the weekends. So she's on stage and goes, 'Hi, I'm your drummer.' She's goofing around with me and I go like, 'Oh really? Well, I'm Bruce' and I'm checking out my guitars and I said something like, 'I hope they behave tonight.' The fact that I treated the guitars kind of like a woman in a way, like my babies, that really turned her on and of course I was flirting with her. She mentioned that on our first date: 'When you said you wanted your guitars to behave that was a big turn-on.' Now, I could never plan something like that. I said it off the cuff; I didn't say it to turn her on.

I remember one time asking a girl: it was at the end of the night after a show and there was a girl that was fairly attractive and she was by herself and I said, 'Who do you belong to?' In a way, I was just like saying, 'I don't have a chance. You're too good-looking to be available' and that's just what came off my tongue. And in the end, she wasn't with anybody, she *loved* that of course because it made her feel attracted and we got to date for a little bit from that. So I know there are guys who always have lines. I would always hear one of my Union bandmates say something silly like, 'I'm going to lick you like a postage stamp,' which to me is not the best way to break the ice with a girl. I always find that any girl I've ever met, there's been some natural kind of thing that I say that kind of makes them unique to what was happening at that moment. That kind of approach, that sincerity of just showing them that you're aware of their social environment, whether it be on stage or in the club… if I'm doing any kind of event and fans know who I am and they meet me, what kind of pick-up line can you say to them? If they let you know they're available, you can just say, 'Hey, what are you doing later?' That's no pick-up line. You know they came to see you and if you're going to spend some time with them they're going to be thrilled – that's part of the joy of being a rock star. I use that loosely, but obviously your typical guy can't get away with that but clearly successful people do. Doctors and lawyers are pretty popular with the women too because they have that kind of power and success. A lot of that is the biggest turn-on for women.

CHIP Z'NUFF: You'd think I'd have them down by this time, but I don't
have any lines. Just come out and be honest, and be kind and sweet, and not disrespectful. If you start the conversation, you've got a chance. My philosophy with women is they're like kitty cats. You hold a kitty cat, you pat it, you kiss it, you hug it and love it, but if you squeeze it too tight eventually it's going to scratch you and bite you and run away. If you use that, you've got a good chance of meeting some nice people. Nobody wants to be smothered unless the time is right. I recommend being kind, although I know there are a few rock musicians (without mentioning any names) who would beg to differ, but my approach has always worked pretty well for me.

COURTNEY TAYLOR-TAYLOR: I'm not good at raunchy. It doesn't come
naturally for me – raunchy being too filthy. For me, it's always just kind of been chat and either I get raped or I don't get laid. I've always been a book-worm, kind of… and I've always been so distracted by music. It is everywhere you are. We need water to survive and you can't get it in your car, but you can get music. If you're in a shopping mall or a supermarket, it could take you ten minutes to get water but there's music around you all the time, constantly. So I've always had pretty bad social skills because I've always been distracted by bad music, good music – good music, I'm just completely phased-out. I've walked out of existence and you can't expect me to hear anything that you just said to me. With bad music it's less, because I'm wondering why the hell this is on and it's been that way since I was about six years old. I've always missed out on anything you could get as a young person by verbal social manipulation. I didn't get it; I missed out on it bad. So the sex thing falls into that.

DANKO JONES: I suck at those. I have none. It doesn't work for me; it just
doesn't. I'm horrible at it. I don't have like a zinger that gets everybody every time. I have nothing.

DOUG ROBB: I'm probably not well known for my pick-up lines. I think being
as charming as I can be is the only way I'd go about it. This girl approached me once and asked me if she could give me a blowjob in the bathroom, with her boyfriend standing right there, and I was like, 'Are you fucking serious? Are you fucking kidding me?' and she was like, 'Oh, it's OK. He doesn't care.' That's an interesting pick-up line!

EVAN SEINFELD: In a world where people expect lines and they expect
bullshit, I've always stuck to a straightforward approach: unlike scripted reality shows, true reality where I've been known to walk up to a girl and say, 'You are so attractive; I really want to have sex with you.' That's my 'line'. And you know

what, the kind of dudes that tell girls bullshit are so weak; they're always like the weakest dudes in the world. There's a particular rock star that I know who lives in LA who mass-texts all these girls that he's thinking about them. That's so utterly gay. My rule is never to pretend it's more than it is; never to act like I'm more interested in a girl than I am. I mean, I'm married; I don't get very interested. So in terms of pick-up lines, I'm that kind of guy who walks right up and says, 'I want to be inside you right now' or 'I really want to hurt you.' If they know what I mean we're usually having sex within minutes. If they don't understand or don't get it, then there wasn't a match there in the first place. More times than not – I'm not a lying kind of person – there's an energy and there's an unspoken language, like a, 'C'mon let's go.' My line is usually, 'Come with me.'

HANDSOME DICK MANITOBA: I don't have those, I'm not that slick. I just don't have those. If I like a girl, I've come to this conclusion that you look at her right in the eye and you just talk to her and that's the sexiest thing in the world. People are in bars, people are in a place where that's what they're doing there and you don't have to have an automated pilot system. You can actually be in the moment and actually just say something and actually mean it and talk. We're already putting females up on a pedestal: the sexual success of man is based on what women I can get and how I can conquer them and everything. There's no rush; you don't have to jump in with a line. There's a lot of women in the world, there's three billion women in the world, or whatever. So some bad lines could work but I ain't that kind of player. I like to really just connect with someone and talk to them and that's it; I don't need a line.

JAMES KOTTAK: 'Hey man, I'm in a rock band.' That always works.

AN OPENING LINE SHOULD REALLY BE A LURE. THAT'S ALL IT IS. IT'S AN INVITATION; IT SHOULD MAKE IT EASY TO WANT TO COME IN.

JESSE HUGHES: 'Have you ever been to heaven?' Nah, I'm just kidding. That actually never works; I want to make that clear. Try looking at someone sometimes if they have a foul look on their face and going, 'This place sucks' and then turning around. That stuff has worked. An opening line should really be a lure. That's all it is. It's an invitation; it should make it easy to want to come in. Being standard doesn't in any way improve your chances, it just makes you standard. If you're actually trying to pick up someone, you'll pick up on them, but if you actually want to get laid, then that's a different game.

JIMMY ASHHURST: We've been playing to a lot of younger crowds these days and the old, 'We've got beer on the bus' seems to be working like a charm, as ridiculous as it is. It never ceases to amaze me how successful that one is. I've also noticed in some of the hotels now they have the Sleep Number beds. There's a commercial on in the States that asks you what your Sleep Number is. I've discovered that mine is a 35, so I've been enjoying going around to ladies saying, 'I know my Sleep Number, do you want to find out yours?' That's a good American one at the moment.

JOEL O'KEEFFE: Anything funny works.

LEMMY: I never know until the moment. 'Do you live around here often?' is quite good. 'Hi. So you want to fuck or what?'

ROB PATTERSON: None. I hate pick-up lines.

TOBY RAND: 'Are you having fun yet?' That's my pick-up line: 'Are you having fun yet?' Whatever response you get, you can go from there.

VAZQUEZ: I can remember the first time I went to LA and I was really excited 'cause it's like you read all these books and see these movies and it was the first time I ever came to LA. I went to the Viper Room and at the time Metal Skool were playing there. So I was on a high and had never been to California before. I'm seeing Metal Skool, who were just fucking great, and I see this gorgeous, gorgeously sick girl – just beautiful! She's walking out of the bathroom and I just look at her and I didn't say anything; I just put my arms out to give her a hug. And the next thing you know, we're back at the Holiday Inn in my manager's bathroom just going fucking crazy.

What pick-up line should be avoided at all costs?

ACEY SLADE: 'Nice shoes.'

BLASKO: I think *all* pick-up lines should be avoided at all costs.

CHIP Z'NUFF: 'I'm new in town. Can you give me your address?' That's an old line from a famous rock singer. It worked for him a few times though. I just wouldn't be too disrespectful.

JAMES KOTTAK: 'So, what's going on?' That's about as boring as you can get.

JIMMY ASHHURST: 'Your friend is hot!'

JOEL O'KEEFFE: 'I would look good in you!'

LEMMY: 'So, you fuck then or what?' Not that that should be avoided at all costs.

NICKE BORG: 'Can I look at your tattoos?'

ROB PATTERSON: 'What's your sign?' That's the worst!

TOBY RAND: 'How do you like your eggs in the morning?'

VAZQUEZ: Well honestly I'm not sure because I think I'm just so gorgeous and so non-threatening to women that pretty much anything I say, no matter how foul it is, they're gonna laugh. I get away with murder man; I don't know why.

What is the best way to guarantee a 'yes' to a date offer?

ACEY SLADE: If it's the girl and she's trying to pick up a guy, the one that always works is, 'Where's your bus?' The one that should be avoided though is, 'Hey, I know your tour manager.' If she knows your tour manager or the crew, it means she's been around. As soon as I see she's buddies with the tour manager or one of the crew, I know that clearly means she's spent a lot of time with other bands.

DANKO JONES: I'm really bad at that. I need to have the girl telegraph me that she's interested. I walk around not knowing. I don't know. I honestly have no clue. I always assume they are not interested so I need it telegraphed to me. That's to my detriment. Over the years I've realised, 'Oh man, I could have had her, I could have been with her. I didn't know she was interested.' It comes to light later, so I have no idea. I walk around assuming that people I'm interested in would not be interested in me.

JOEL O'KEEFFE: 'I'm buying, so what have you got to lose?'

ROB PATTERSON: There is no way; everyone is different.

TOBY RAND: A guaranteed yes is if you tell a girl, 'We're going to go and have a shitload of fucking fun' and nothing else.

Where is an ideal place to go for a first date?

ACEY SLADE: New York, just in general. I'm a good New York tour guide. That's my backyard and I know a ton of places to show someone. So it's nice to have home turf advantage.

ADDE: To a King Diamond concert, which is my favourite band. If she can stand me after that then that's the match made in heaven right there.

ALLISON ROBERTSON: I'm actually really into food, so if they took me to one of my favourite Mexican restaurants… I love when a guy can read my mind and I don't have to ask them what they want and they actually like the same things. An ideal first date would be if they said they wanted to watch my favourite movie but they didn't know it was my favourite movie, and just go get some good Mexican food or a pizza. I'm really easy. I'm actually so easy it's sad. I just really like someone who you can do normal things with *and* go out and do something crazy with. Either way it's the same and it's always sexy and it's always comfortable. To me, there's like a balance that's really hard to find there.

ANDREW W.K.: I always thought that the first date should always end in making out and sex. I don't know why I ever got that idea but for that reason, I guess going over to the girl's house or having her come straight to your house for the first date isn't something that I think is too crazy. I guess you want to go to the restaurant first, but the idea is to always wind up there. I think that's what both people are thinking about whether they want to do it or not. To me, the idea of going to a restaurant or going to a movie, or getting together with friends, that doesn't even count as the date so much because really those are just sort of ramping up, primers to get to someone's house. So really, the first date is all about getting there and that's when you really learn the most about that person also. I think it's only fair and acceptable to want to see that other person's house; how they live, where they live, what their room looks like. That to me is probably going to be more important than anything I could learn from dinner if I want to be intimate with a person.

BLASKO: I suppose generally speaking, places that are standard. I mean, shit dude, I've been married for a long time so I'm kind of out of the loop. I would say the restaurant – dinner is kind of standard and always kind of works.

BRENT MUSCAT: When I was living in LA there was a hotel downtown and there was a restaurant on the very top floor that rotated 360 degrees, so you could just sit there and within an hour it would spin you all around downtown LA and you could see everywhere. On a clear night you could see the ocean, you could see mountains. That was one of my favourite spots in LA. That was one of my secret spots. It was great because you could just go up there and have a drink too. It wasn't like you had to eat; you could just go up for a drink. It's called the Bona Vista Lounge.

BRUCE KULICK: I know a movie is a horrible thing. I really think getting together over a casual meal is fun or doing something together that would be either your interest or her interest and see how that goes. For me, I'd love to take a girl to a guitar show or even a store and show her, 'This is my hobby. This is my life. These are fun things.' Now, I'm not necessarily saying that's exciting for the girl but I even don't mind, 'Well let's grab a little bite or a cup of coffee and walk around the boulevard.' There's always a place to window-shop and walk around and then you get to see… I had a disastrous date with a porno star once who expressed interest in me at this Kiss Expo that I did. The fact that she showed any interest in me to begin with was pretty shocking. Obviously, when I'd tell a friend they're like, 'Oh my God! You're going to have a date with her?' I didn't know if I wanted to have a date with her and I didn't know if I wanted to fuck her because I'm intimidated by that. I want to make my own porn movie with a girl-next-door that is a real person and not a real professional. A stripper doesn't turn me on because I know it's a game; they're only carrying on because they want money. So anyway, what was a good, easy thing to do? 'Third Street Promenade in Santa Monica; meet you there!' Food, shopping, walking; I even took my dog as an ice-breaker. As much as she was almost as crazy as I expected, I'm glad I didn't take it any further because I couldn't spend five minutes really comfortably with her. It's one thing to see that she's hot and another thing to know that she knows how to fuck the shit out of any guy. That's not really going to do it for me. I need some kind of connection as a human being. I'm not saying she was a bad person, it's just I'm not going to connect with her and I know it – so that was the end of that. She probably got the sense that I just wasn't for her either, but even if she wanted to take it further I don't think I would have. In one way you could say, 'You're going to pass up this hot chick?' but yeah, if I'm not going to feel really comfortable, I don't want to deal with it. There's always going to be something that bites you in the ass afterwards about it.

CHIP Z'NUFF: I've got to be honest with you: I think a great restaurant would be terrific to start the ball rolling. However, a lot of these girls I meet, they all love movies so maybe take her to the Cinemax. Go to a nice IMAX theatre; watch a flick together, that's good. Remember the old drive-in movies where you pay your comp, drive in and roll your window down and put the speakers in there? If you can get her in the drive-in theatre, you'll get the ball rolling for sure. If she's going to go to the drive-in theatre with you, there's obviously something about you that trips her trigger, so that's probably your best bet.

COURTNEY TAYLOR-TAYLOR: An ideal place for a first date is like a downtown (gay part of downtown) coffee shop where you've got kind of edgy to straight-up derelict people to trendy kids – just a good overall blend of everything, where you can just see how they look at other people and how you feel about them in that situation. Are they uncomfortable, are they comfortable? Are they excited or are they overly excited? Are they intimidated? And mostly, will they eat a piece of cheesecake and drink coffee at ten o'clock at night? Or do they have little dietary issues? Because that's something you do a lot; you go eat a lot together. How do they deal with wait staff? How do they deal with things going wrong with what they ordered? Or needing an extra fork? All that stuff. I think that's the most perfect and I did that religiously as a high school student all the way up through. I always have. It's never failed me. Really, until I started dating outside of my own town and ending up some place where I just started to have real fuck-ups, real embarrassing situations like, 'How did I get myself into this?' Or, 'It's a stalker,' or, 'This person is crazy.' I never had that problem at home because being a very young, downtown musician kid at like 14/15 years old, I'd end up with some girl that I liked and she liked me. So I'd just take them out like that until they finally make a pass at you or don't.

DANKO JONES: I always do a very generic thing: dinner is always a very good way of getting to know somebody. I'm talking about somebody you're actually very interested in as a person. I'm not talking about any one-night stand thing. With someone you're genuinely interested in and you see a possibility of taking it to the next level, it's as simple as dinner. Or even coffee. I don't really put any elaborate plans into it. I know other people do. I'm bad at that. So my best bet is to just have dinner and get to know the person. If it sucks, then you just go, 'Well I've got to go, thanks for dinner. Bye!'

DOUG ROBB: A strip club? I don't know who would take their first date to a strip club but that would probably set the tone.

EVAN SEINFELD: Me personally, when I was single, if I was dating to find a girlfriend I would take girls off to the same place, either the same restaurant or the same club. I like to take girls to a gentleman's club on the first date to ensure that they're not uptight; they're not uptight about other girls and make sure they're not insecure, because insecure girls talk shit about all the girls, like, 'Oh, she's fat; she's ugly' or, 'What a skank' and I'm immediately turned off. But if they flirt with the other girls and they enjoy the moment, then I'm super turned on. I kind of use it as a great barometer to take their temperature.

GINGER: A park. If you can't find enough to keep conversation going amid nature then you can call it quits and say goodbye. Avoid eating in front of each other until the second date. It can be uncomfortable and you don't want to be stuck at dinner with someone you can't communicate with. Remember it's OK not to hit it off with someone on a date. It always pays to be completely honest with your emotions.

HANDSOME DICK MANITOBA: My ideal first date is not a pre-fab first date too much. It's not a good idea to go to a movie because you're just sitting side-by-side looking at something else and it's not a good idea to go eat immediately because eating is like a personal thing. It's sounds and chewing; it's kind of an animalistic thing. You don't necessarily want to share that immediately. So in my history, my idea of a perfect date has always been, 'Hey, let's get together and take a walk.' Spend 15 minutes and talk and take a walk, then as you're connecting you say, 'Let's go _____' and then you go do it. You work your way up to eat, work your way up to going to a movie, work your way up to going to a park.

JAMES KOTTAK: A good place to go? Of course a rock concert, because you don't have to talk to each other.

JESSE HUGHES: It depends on the girl. You always have to consider the subject. An ideal place for a first date can be a place her Daddy never took her.

JIMMY ASHHURST: Anywhere that's away from a rock'n'roll environment; some place where you can actually understand what the person is saying. It's been like 20 years for me now of going like, 'What?' back and forth, which is great, but you often discover too late that you haven't really understood a word of what she's said the entire time you've been together… which is also great sometimes. If I'm home and in town, then a great restaurant is always the move.

JOEL O'KEEFFE: The bar because a) you both get drunk, which will loosen her defences up, and b) if she's not 'up for it' then you still get drunk and there's plenty of other now-gorgeous options available. Everyone is a winner!

LEMMY: Well, it used to be the pictures, didn't it? We used to go to the movies but movies are so miserable now it's not worth it. A restaurant's nice; a nice meal.

NICKE BORG: Since I'm such a sucker for good wine and food, I'd recommend taking the person to a great restaurant with great fucking wine and food. To enjoy that as much as you probably would later on enjoy whatever you're planning to do, that's… I think there's something really, really sexy about someone who appreciates good wine and food with you.

ROB PATTERSON: Starbucks?

TOBY RAND: First date for me would be something really casual: go and see a band, or go to a beer garden and have a few drinks and then sit on the beach, have a few more drinks, and just kiss… Or if it's in the snow you just fuck, don't ya? Go for a snowboard then sit by the fire.

VAZQUEZ: Ideally, it would be my house… But I don't really do dates; that's not how I roll. You know, I'll meet a girl and we'll hang out, maybe take a ride on the motorcycle or something like that.

How important is personality versus appearance?

ACEY SLADE: It depends on what you're looking for: I'm at a stage in my life where personality is everything. Obviously they have to be attractive in some capacity. I've been with some extremely beautiful women who are very, very shallow. If you're looking to get laid, that's great but for actually taking someone on a date and actually spending time with someone, personality is most important, for sure.

ADDE: Oh the personality is everything. I don't really go that much on the face and everything like that. Personality is way more important!

BLASKO: Initially appearance, and then personality. I mean, look at it this way: I've never got onto an ugly chick and then realised after I talked to her that she was really cool. Like, that has never happened. But I've certainly got on many a hot chick and realised they were a total cunt afterwards and wanted nothing to do with them.

YOU CAN BE A KNOCKOUT BUT IF YOU OPEN YOUR MOUTH AND AIR COMES OUT, THAT WILL ONLY LAST SO LONG.

DOUG ROBB: It's pretty important. You can be a knockout but if you open your mouth and air comes out, that will only last so long. As far as flings, personality doesn't weigh in at all; it's all just appearance. But if you want to spend any amount of time with somebody, personality weighs much heavier, if not as heavy, as their appearance.

JOEL O'KEEFFE: Well, they're both really important… but then again, you're not making small talk or looking at the mantle piece when you're stoking the fire are you?

ROB PATTERSON: It is the most important thing. You can only look at someone for so long before they start speaking.

TOBY RAND: Lately I've discovered that personality is of the utmost importance… although I love looking at girls at the same time.

How do you know when dating has become more serious and you are actually a couple?

ACEY SLADE: Probably when she asks you to get a job.

ALLISON ROBERTSON: Yeah, that's hard to know. When you're a girl you don't want to push to find that out, so I feel like I don't know unless they actually say, 'Do you want to be my girlfriend?' I think it's fair to assume that if somebody is with you all the time and either of you are not dating other people or whatever that you're probably a couple, but some people don't feel comfortable with that. To me, I don't really assume it until it's said… and there's a signed contract.

ANDREW W.K.: I think when the idea of being with someone else isn't appealing. You can still go on dates and still be seeing other people, but when you finish the date with this one person and you find yourself not wanting to leave or wanting to go back the next day or not wanting to hang out with that other girl, then it's become more serious.

BLASKO: I think you just know.

BRENT MUSCAT: When you start getting jealous. When you start getting jealous feelings, you know that you have something. Or when you start getting those feelings of worrying who they're out with, or where they're at, wondering what they're doing. I think when you start getting those kinds of feelings you've grown attached.

BRUCE KULICK: If you're speaking every day, and you want some company and you're thinking of that person, that's when you're really not single any more. It's time to just hone in on that person and just know if that person is worthy of all that energy from me instead of just playing the field.

CHIP Z'NUFF: It's usually pretty self-explanatory. The woman, just by how she carries herself, will tell you. If she says, 'I've had such a wonderful time. I can't wait to see you again' that means you've won. Or, 'I'll call you later' is another sign. I think the old rule of thumb of, 'Don't call a girl for a couple of days afterwards' is bullshit. You always want to be respected. It's always nice to call and say, 'Hey, how you doing?' without being smothering of course. Just calling to make sure they're OK. I think that's a nice thing to do too. It's very important to be thoughtful. Little gifts don't hurt either, and not just flowers because that's boring. A little FedEx gift of something nice, something special, has always seemed to work for most of my friends.

COURTNEY TAYLOR-TAYLOR: Well obviously there are a lot of ways, like the first time she says, 'Hey!' about you talking to some other girl too long or when you're rubbing your shoulders with some other girl that you are old friends with and maybe had a mutual crush on, never got it together, got it together and you let her rub your shoulders still because otherwise it would hurt her feelings or something. You know, just some weird shit you do between girlfriends and you let a lot happen, like when her arm is around you when they're talking with someone else, like you're buddies. It's a girl and you're a guy – you're buddies. There's the first time for a lot of things. So, when she says, 'Oh, great. I'm going to be in Europe around then' and then when you come back she had been in Europe for two months staying in your apartment so she's just staying at your house now. That's when you know you're a couple.

DANKO JONES: That's a very grey line; I don't know myself. I've been out on dates with girls, like you go out maybe four or five times, and I don't consider that girlfriend-boyfriend and they have in the past. So there's been mixed signals I guess. I don't think four or five dates is enough for you to go, 'OK, well we're boyfriend-girlfriend now.' I just think it's more of a feel. Both parties feel.

DOUG ROBB: I think maybe when you start to think about the person you are 'dating' and if you can picture them with another person and you're like, 'Oh whatever. I could still go out and hook up with other girls', then you're just dating. But if you get to the point where you think about the person you're with being with another person and it makes you a little uncomfortable and a little mad, I think you probably have some investment in there.

EVAN SEINFELD: When that person becomes a priority over new pussy; when you've got the option between strange pussy and the woman you're seeing, and your option is to see the woman.

HANDSOME DICK MANITOBA: I don't know. The girl will let you know. Girls are in charge of relationships; she'll tell you.

JAMES KOTTAK: When she's paying for dinner.

JESSE HUGHES: When you start deleting text messages from your phone right before you get home.

JIMMY ASHHURST: When you start getting shit about your MySpace comments.

JOEL O'KEEFFE: If you find yourself chasing her by flying out to meet her between shows and she's doing the same for you, it's hook, line and sinker for you two. Or the other less costly but more violent one is when she catfights with your real girlfriend – then you are in the shit big time! It's in these times that you are very thankful for the mobile safety bubble factor of the tour bus to take you far away to a new paradise where you can start afresh again.

THE CHASE IS BETTER THAN THE CATCH IS WHAT THEY SAY AND THEY'RE RIGHT.

LEMMY: When her father knocks on the door with the shotgun barrels. I don't know; it's individual – you know that. Usually only one of you feels it anyway. It's always one chasing the other, more or less. I mean, it changes within the relationship. It can change from one being chased, you turn around and the one being chased becomes the chaser. It's weird like that. I'm sure you all know what I'm talking about. The chase is better than the catch is what they say and they're right.

ROB PATTERSON: You just know. For example, when you go on tour and your heart aches when I am not with my fiancée.

TOBY RAND: When you go out to a pub or a club and your partner's not with you and you go home by yourself – that's how you know.

VAZQUEZ: Oh man, that's real easy: as soon as they start screaming at you for no reason, you're in a relationship!

DIVORCE

"BUT ONCE YOU START HAVING A SHIT WHILE YOUR GIRL BRUSHES HER TEETH - THAT'S TIME TO GET A DIVORCE"

When do you know it's time to get a divorce?

ACEY SLADE: When she tells another guy in your band that she married you for a green card.

ADDE: When they don't appreciate you for who you are. When they try to bring you down because of who you are.

ALLISON ROBERTSON: I've been divorced. To me, what leads to divorce, in my head, is feeling too comfortable. I think you have to balance between being comfortable and having excitement. I think that's the rare thing that people can't really ever find. You're really excited about somebody but then it gets boring, or you're always excited but then everybody's always cheating on each other and it's not really very stable. For marriage, if you get too comfortable and there's no fun going on, that usually leads to divorce. Either that or fighting a lot, but in my case it was too comfortable and not enough excitement to keep it looking good in the future.

ANDREW W.K.: I don't know and I hope I never do, but just from relationships that might as well have been marriages, breaking up is like a divorce. But see, it's different: being married is not just like being in a committed relationship. It has a power to it because you made a decision, I made a decision, and the idea is to make a decision based on eternity. That's a very different headspace. Even if you don't think that way, just to have engaged in something where that is meant to be the understanding changes things. When I was younger I would have thought that the minute you don't enjoy each other's company in the same way or as much, then you should get a divorce. Or if one person cheats on the other person they should get a divorce. Or if they just have no interest in one another. But I've seen marriages go through those things – not my own but other people that have been married for longer – and there's often been this idea that you should never get divorced and you stay together no matter what. When I was younger I thought that was really disturbing, because it seemed like people throwing away their life or throwing away certain opportunities to be happy in a different way; but as I've got older I've also seen that it's extremely brave and that sacrificing certain opportunities and types of happiness for other types that have been considered more valuable, like maintaining a family if you have kids, or maintaining a promise, or working through it with this idea that you committed to it and you can improve it. So there's been so many aspects to the concept of marriage that have seemed unnatural, that have seemed to go against the reproductive urges, that have seemed to go against this logic of the idea that two people can remain the same in a way that allows them to be connected to the same way as they were at one point throughout their whole lives. It seems crazy, but at the same time that's why it's powerful because you are choosing to do something that is untraditionally challenging and is unusually powerfully committing. But I think that's the whole point: the fact that in theory we can go and have sex with anybody we want is why it's powerful to not do it. You turn that energy towards the relationship or towards yourself or towards this partnership with another person and that's really the concept.

BRENT MUSCAT: I've never got one, so I don't know.

BRUCE KULICK: As my therapist would say… obviously a real relationship is going to have some bumps in the road; you have to have that – that's what's real. The people who always act like everything's hunky dory, that's the one who always gets blindsided the worst, so I find that one of the signals would be when they hit you below the belt. I don't mean physically of course; obviously if they're hitting you, you've got to run for the hills. When someone says something to you that's so hurtful and unfair, and as my therapist would say, 'It's below the belt', those things can never be taken back. Now, I'm not saying the first time you hear one of those you've got to get divorced. First you've got to call your partner out on it; they've got to know they hit below the belt and that you're not going to accept that again and don't go there if you want a relationship to last. I can't even give you an example of what's hitting below the belt, but you know it. It's different for everybody. It's about pushing a button of what makes you tick and if someone can say something so hurtful to you, that's what that is – certainly something you wouldn't say to a friend, you know? If you're a lover and your partner's supposed to be your best friend, then why would you say that? But unfortunately that's what happens in relationships. They say we're acting out, trying to correct our parents' relationship; there's all this psychology behind it – who knows? But I know, as soon as I've heard a few of those things, I'd be like, 'I don't want to be married to this person in the future.'

CHIP Z'NUFF: I knew the day I got married. I got married in Las Vegas. The first time I got married it was terrific. I married my high school sweetheart. We had a great run; however I was on tour all the time. Enuff Z'Nuff were very successful and we were travelling all around the country and she found another friend, which was drugs, and that's usually a killer on every relationship – substance abuse. You try and make it work for the first however much time you put into it – six months, a year, whatever – that they're trying to get clean, but the percentages always say it's not going to work. That didn't work and I got married again three, four or five years later. I got married to my second wife and the day I got married, it was a perfect day for a marriage. I was in Las Vegas out on tour with this band called The Wild Bunch. It was Clem Burke from Blondie, Wayne Kramer from MC5, Pat from The Smithereens, Gilby Clarke; the girls in The Go-Gos were there and just all these rock stars hanging out. It was just a perfect time. They all wanted to come of course, so they came to the wedding and the day I'm at the wedding, I looked at the camera and said, 'I'm doomed!'

I knew it. I could just feel it. It was much better just staying boyfriend-girlfriend, but she insisted on my undivided attention and I gave into her on a whim. I knew that day I was doomed and I went seven years longer just drenched and clothed in pain. So for anybody out there thinking about getting married, you'd better make sure this is the right thing because I don't know anybody that gets married for a failure. However, I failed twice.

COURTNEY TAYLOR-TAYLOR: It is time to get a divorce when you first see a problem in their behaviour that you really honestly deep in your heart of hearts know you can't tolerate for the rest of your life. When you think about it for the rest of your life, you want to die. You really, really do. You really do. You just go, 'OK, even if it's just once a year. No. It's going to get worse. Twice a year? It's already up to twice a year. Oh my God' and you just go, 'OK, if I could just not behave like this. I want to make sure she's not in that situation. I don't put her in that situation. If she starts it in public I'm not even going to react to it.' When you've done that, when you've done everything you can do, including admitting fault for it and taking the blame for it yourself to kind of fix it on your own end and it's been a year, a couple of years, like three years and it's just like, 'Fuck. I fucked up. I didn't know… She faked me out. We dated for four years and she's pulled that shit.' So that's when you know it's time to divorce. So, what it's really time to do is to not be facing each other when you have this conversation, hopefully both be lying down on a sofa or a love-seat, not within reach of each other and not facing or looking at each other's face when you have this conversation. You have to tell them that you don't know if you can live with this, like, 'I've been nice every day and it's been fun, but you've probably noticed I haven't been as touchy, huggy, kissy with you and stuff and I've just got to tell you that I've come to the realisation that I'm not going to be able to live with this for the rest of my life and I'd rather we just end this now so we can both move on and get it over. It'll be rough for a year, year and a half, but then we'll be happy and free.' The other person gets pissed off, or completely calmly says, 'Yeah, I'm not going to change that about myself' and that's it, or gets pissed off and can't handle talking about that part of themselves and four hours later doesn't calm down. If that impasse is real for you and you've tried, that is exactly when you know. You very painfully and calmly deal with it and do the open-heart surgery or whatever it takes. Just get through it, get beyond it. A divorce is just like breaking up a serious, long-term relationship. I've had girlfriends longer and more substantial and serious relationships than probably most marriages. So divorce or breaking up is all the same, except maybe the legal shit of it later in life.

DANKO JONES: Oh God, I'm bad at that too. I have a real tendency to just beat a dead horse – not literally. What I mean is I'll stay until the very, very end. I'm really bad at that, so what ends up happening is I'm the one that ends up getting dumped because the girl is just going, 'Don't you know? Are you going to do it or am I going to have to do it?' So they always have to do it because I just don't. I'm always like, 'Oh we can fix this.' I'm like one of those kinds of people.

DOUG ROBB: I have no idea. I'm recently married, about eight months ago, and I hope I never find out.

EVAN SEINFELD: I've been divorced. I think intuitively, we know. I think it's a matter of getting honest with ourselves about it. And I know for me, or when there's children involved, everybody needs like a therapist or a mentor or a sounding board where they can talk to people and kind of hear themselves talk. Ultimately, I think we have all of our answers and I think once we get to the point where we need to make a list of pros and cons to weigh up whether we should stay in the relationship or not any more, I think it's time to move on. If you need to go there, you're out of there.

GINGER: When communication ends. When you stop learning from each other. When you stop inspiring each other. When honesty is lost. You can work on anything but dishonesty.

HANDSOME DICK MANITOBA: I have never been divorced but I would say when the friendship, communication and respect goes out the window. It's a very tough thing. You're really asking for your mate to be (well, I am anyway) a wild sexual partner and a buddy, a friend. If any of those major things gets off the track then it's trouble signs.

JAMES KOTTAK: When her boyfriend's jackets don't fit you any more.

JESSE HUGHES: Well, like in my case when your ex-wife moves out a house full of furniture, it might be a clue. But it's time to get a divorce when all you're really doing in the relationship is trying to get equity with someone else. And never marry someone whose parents aren't married.

JIMMY ASHHURST: I wouldn't know; I've never been in that situation. I've tried valiantly to avoid it, so I really wouldn't know.

LEMMY: I've never been married you see, so I'll have to exit that one. But probably when your wife lays out the mushrooms and they're all red with white spots on them. You know that joke: this guy says, 'I've been unlucky in love mate. I've been married twice and they've both died. The first one died from eating poison mushrooms.' The other guy says, 'Oh yeah. What did the second one die of?' and he says, 'A blow to the head.' 'How did that happen?' 'She wouldn't eat her mushrooms.'

NICKE BORG: Hopefully there would not be such a time, but I think that depends on person to person. But once you start having a shit while your girl brushes her teeth – that's time to get a divorce.

ROB PATTERSON: When your wife is fucking some other dude.

VAZQUEZ: I've never been married but I've definitely had my share of relationships. This is going to sound totally crazy but when it stops being all about me, then I'm ready to go. That's what happens. Like, these girls go, 'Oh but it's not all about you' and I go, 'No honey, that's really cute and everything that you think that, but it is all about me. Me, me, me.'

If your partner wants a divorce, should you try and talk them out of it?

ACEY SLADE: I think that you should stick to it, by all means necessary. I don't think that therapy is for pussies because I think it can be good to have a third person – there are three sides to every story: there's your side, their side and the truth. But, I think that when your partner says something like, 'Therapy is for pussies' and won't commit to that, then it's time.

ADDE: No, no. That's gone too far already. If you're talking like that, just rip it off.

ALLISON ROBERTSON: Well that depends how much you think you could change. I've seen people change. I'm not talking from my own place but I think it's possible to fix a marriage. If it's not mutual and one person wants the divorce, I think so long as you talk about it and maybe if they have a reason why, you fix it. But if somebody just doesn't want to be with you, I think it's kind of humiliating to try to make them stay.

BRENT MUSCAT: Yeah I do. You should try to work it out as much as you can, especially if you have kids and stuff. I think it's better for the kids to have a mum and a dad both around preferably, and I just think that if people were good enough friends and lovers to get married in the first place, I think that they could still stay together. Even if the marriage isn't working, I don't think it would hurt to be partners and stay together for a while and share the household. Even if they were like room-mates, you know. I think you can find common ground where you can give it a chance to rekindle the fire or rekindle the love.

BRUCE KULICK: I think the only way that you'd have a chance to reverse that is to try some counselling. I don't think it's a bad thing. I have tried it and what's really interesting is usually a lot of the stuff that is just stuck under the rug will certainly spring to life and at worst things might just be clearer for both of you on why you shouldn't be together. Of course if there's children involved...

financially it's devastating for any couple, so it's worth it to explore that, but usually when someone's that upset to file, you could very well be in the condition red already and you may not be able to reverse it.

CHIP Z'NUFF: You should talk about it, absolutely. Talk them out of it? No. But talk about it. It's important to express your feelings. To hold and suppress that in is just like a cancer; it's just going to eat you away. So yeah, you talk about it but if they want to get out, my Gramps said, 'Let the bird fly. If it comes back to you, you know it was meant to be. If it doesn't, that's it.' I think for a guy or a woman who's just smothering and can't stand the thought of not being with that person, if they need time away in a separation from you, I think you should grant that wish. In more times than others, it'll come back to you where it'll be good and you'll realise that that little time of separation away cleansed yourself.

IT'S IMPORTANT TO EXPRESS YOUR FEELINGS. TO HOLD AND SUPPRESS THAT IN IS JUST LIKE A CANCER; IT'S JUST GOING TO EAT YOU AWAY.

DANKO JONES: Yeah I have, definitely. Over the years though I've come to realise that if one person wants out then it should be finished immediately. It took me a while; it has to do with maturity. You've got to go through life and you've got to go through things a few times and then you realise every single relationship you've had… if you're a sane person you evaluate your relationship when it's finished and you go, 'Well what did I do wrong? OK, that really bothered the other person. I'm going to work on that and not do that again. What is it about that person that drove me up the wall? Well I'm going to watch out for that trait and I'm going to be aware of it and I'm not going to fall into a pattern.' Some people are like, 'Oh, I like this girl because she reminds me of my ex-girlfriend' and then people just go into these patterns and nothing changes. So that's what I have done with myself, because the first time it happened I was really hurt and I was like, 'Well what the fuck is wrong with me?' so I really started to develop that habit.

EVAN SEINFELD: Your partner wants a divorce because it's something tangible. You should always try to resolve it if you've got time and energy invested into the relationship because sometimes people are looking to get a divorce because they're afraid of being in love, because they might get hurt because they've been hurt before. And it might be for what might happen, rather than what's wrong. So I always think it's worth talking out. Once you invest time or energy into something you should always try to see it through; don't bail at the first sign. Relationships are not easy; they're very hard, very complicated. Men and women want very different things in marriages. If I had to boil it down in a nutshell, women use sex to get love, men use love to get sex. It's like doing a dance; it looks completely symbiotic but it's not.

HANDSOME DICK MANITOBA: I think you should be involved enough in your own life and relationship to know what's going on. There shouldn't be shock at what's going on or else you might be pulling the wool over your own eyes in advance.

JAMES KOTTAK: No, go for it. Get it over with, move on. As we say, especially if it's your first marriage in Los Angeles, we call that your starter marriage.

JESSE HUGHES: Of course, especially if you have children. The benefit of marriage to the spirit and to the other spiritual aspects of human health is beyond simply the person you're with. It's the commitment and sticking with something through your life as an institution; that's where the benefit lies. We've forgotten that and we've devalued that, so of course, I tried to talk mine out of it even though I hated her.

JIMMY ASHHURST: Absolutely not! I think if it's gone that far… I've known several people that have tried to live in misery and it's no way to do it. Even if it's for the family, the benefit of the kids, or whatever, if it's not happening you need to make alternative arrangements if it's got to that point.

LEMMY: If it's got to that stage, it's pretty hopeless anyway.

ROB PATTERSON: Absolutely not! You do not own a person – period.

TOBY RAND: No, if they want a divorce then… You can't talk someone into doing something they don't want to do.

VAZQUEZ: I don't think so. I mean, who the fuck would want to be with somebody who doesn't want to be with you?

At what point should you get a lawyer involved if you see divorce looming?

ACEY SLADE: I'll let you know in the next few days.

ALLISON ROBERTSON: If either of you has more money than the other one. I don't think you necessarily have to get a lawyer though. If you've shared everything and you just want to split it you can get someone cheap to come in and keep it equal. Otherwise, it depends how much you're fighting or feelings are mutual. If it's like, 'Hey I don't really like you any more' you might not care about it. It really depends how much money is involved.

BRENT MUSCAT: Never. I got married and somebody said I should get a pre-nup and I'm like, 'Why? I'm not rich. Like, I've got a house and stuff but it's not like I'm a rich guy.' My theory was that if I'm going to get married to someone and she's going to help me and be my partner, then I said if I did get divorced I'd happily give her half. I don't care; it's only money and it's only a material thing. It's like, if the woman's there helping you and she's your partner… With my wife, I was in debt, I was a mess and a wreck (I married her around 2000/2001) and she helped me get my shit together. I would not sign a pre-nup; I would happily give her half of anything I have. So I would just say, 'Be generous and don't get a lawyer, because if you get a lawyer it's just going to cost more money anyway; you're just wasting your money. So save money, give her what she wants.' I mean, if you have to do that and you want to get away, don't be greedy.

BRUCE KULICK: Every country and every state is different. I'll talk about my main divorce from the girl from all my Kiss years because we knew how ugly it could be. I think she even hoped that it would work and it was me that finally said, 'Wait a minute, I'm not going back for more of this. I didn't deserve this' blah, blah, blah. I kind of felt that even though my heart was broken, I didn't know what was on her mind. The counselling certainly didn't help it and I realised once I put myself back together… I want to move on. But the smart thing that we did, as much as she was going to stand her ground, was that we had a lawyer represent both of us, which makes more money go to both of you ultimately, because you're not paying for two different lawyers. Ultimately, I do think that it's different for everybody.

CHIP Z'NUFF: Well if she's fucking the football team then it's time to get a lawyer for sure, because most guys have fragile egos and they can't take that. However, if someone's got a drinking problem or a substance abuse problem and you really love them and you've been with them for years, I believe you should try and work it out. My Gramps told me, he said, 'For every year you're married and you break up, it's one month of pain.' So if you're married to somebody for ten years, expect ten months of pain and there's nothing you can do about it. You can bring new trim into the household, you can try different things, but it's not going to replace the person that tripped your trigger in the first place. So get ready for ten months of pain if you've been married for ten years. Don't hold onto it because it's going to get worse and worse and worse. Be grateful for the time that you spent with that person too OK, because nobody can ever take that away from you. You get to have that. You get to keep the memories – that's free and that's for a lifetime. Good times and great things that happened with you, you'll always be able to look back on that fondly.

COURTNEY TAYLOR-TAYLOR: Before you get married you should really cut your deal, make it clear what you both think you're going into and what is going to be intolerable. Just expect this is real life and go and cut a deal first while you both are positive and feeling as the big person you want to be.

JAMES KOTTAK: If you can avoid the lawyers, do it yourself. Save the money. Just end it, just end it.

JESSE HUGHES: The second you know it's happening. And men, do *not* fall for the oldest trick in the book: you are more than a pay cheque a month. Like, you need a lawyer fast and you need a woman lawyer if you're a man.

ROB PATTERSON: The second you find out something is wrong.

How can assets be best protected in divorce?

ACEY SLADE: In my situation, I'm pretty lucky because I don't have much except for guitars. I'm not a fan of pre-nups; I've always been a fan of only wanting to get married once. Even though I'm a rock'n'roll scumbag on one hand, I'm kind of old-fashioned on the other hand. I'm in the middle of a divorce now, but I only wanted to get married once, so things like pre-nups never really came into my mind.

EVEN THOUGH I'M A ROCK'N'ROLL SCUMBAG ON ONE HAND, I'M KIND OF OLD-FASHIONED ON THE OTHER HAND.

EVAN SEINFELD: Have a pre-nup in the first place. I think it's the nature of women in America to see what they can get out of it. It goes back to my theory that a lot of women are not really into sex for the sex, or the relationship, but more for what they can get out of it. I live in Hollywood man; go down to the Ivy tonight. There's fucking gorgeous 20-year-old Playmates sitting with fucking 80-year-old guys with no teeth. What are they doing there? It's what we call a mutually beneficial relationship; everybody gets something out of this. I don't think that simply because a woman has a vagina and a man has a penis and they try to have a relationship and it doesn't work out then the man has to pay the woman, but unfortunately it's how our society sees it. Women want to be an equal sex, yet the law protects them as the weaker sex.

JESSE HUGHES: Have the bitch killed… kidding. You best protect your assets by being upfront and reasonable and honest and assuming ownership of something. Protecting your assets sometimes means owning it all and you don't necessarily get to do that either if you built something with someone. Especially if there's children involved, sending that message to your kids, 'What would you do if someone spoke bad of your mother?' So you'd better remember that when dealing with the mother of your kids.

JIMMY ASHHURST: Offshore accounts.

ROB PATTERSON: We want pre-nup! ('Gold Digger' by Kayne West.)

DRUGS & ALCOHOL
(& IMPOTENCE)

"TEQUILA USUALLY WORKS WONDERS ON A GIRL'S INHIBITION, BUT NO MORE THAN A SHOT OR TWO"

How can one avoid being flaccid in the sack after a big night out?

ACEY SLADE: I've been sober for 11 years so I don't have that problem. I don't have beer goggles any more either.

ADDE: You just have to take the sexiest girl, you know. If she's ugly in any way, it won't work. I'm sorry, but it won't work.

ALLISON ROBERTSON: I think guys can be better at sex if they're drunk, but I've seen a few that when they drink too much they're barely able to stay awake. So that to me depends on the guy and how much control they have.

ANDREW W.K.: I've actually never been a big drinker so I've not had this problem from alcohol, but there were times when I was just so nervous much earlier on, when I was first being with girls, that sometimes I'd just be so nervous that I couldn't get fully aroused. It was so strange that here was the most stimulating, exciting experience that I had fantasised about through my whole life, here it was actually happening, and I was so revved up in that fact of it happening that it was almost like I wasn't there again. It was like a fantasy all over again. It was so intense and powerful that I experienced moments of impotence. There was so much blood being flushed to my face, my heart was beating so fast that I felt like I couldn't get the blood anywhere else where it was more valued. I've had a few times of being very drunk with sex where I did things I wouldn't have normally done, like not wear a condom. That was disturbing! That was much more disturbing than if I had not been able to perform. I only had that happen the one time. Waking up the next day, I couldn't believe I did it. It felt like it was out of a movie, or out of a TV show or something; the crazy guy who takes this big risk while he's drunk and doesn't realise it and wakes up the next day and had either got a girl pregnant or got some disease or whatever. That was definitely from having drunk a lot of alcohol.

BLASKO: This is probably the best question for Lemmy! I can only say this: the last thing you want to do is put yourself in the position to not put on a show. You kind of know going into it that that's going to be the end result. So you have to go into it kind of minding your P's and Q's. Like, stay away from certain things – know your limitations beforehand.

BRENT MUSCAT: Wait until the morning, get up and have some morning sex. Just brush your teeth, because you'll probably have really bad morning breath.

BRUCE KULICK: I'm not really a drinker and I'm not really a drug-taker. Fortunately, I haven't had that problem. I can say that when I was a teenager and I was in an uncomfortable position sometimes, I thought like, 'This doesn't feel right. I'm going to excuse myself', you know what I mean? Usually I was just really horny and I knew when I wanted to be with somebody. I'll tell you one thing that can affect that: complete exhaustion will affect it. If you've been up for 20 hours working stressful hours, don't expect to have a lot of excitement in the bedroom, especially if the girl wasn't working 20 hours like you just did. Have a good nap then bang her! So, I know that they say, 'Oh, if you drank a lot you can't get it up', but I never drank a lot and the time I did, sadly, I do regret once or twice when I partied too hard and I had a really nice girl that I wanted to have sex with and instead I just got sick. Forget not getting it up; we're talking about praying to the toilet all night, so how am I going to have sex? I regretted that pretty badly. It was like a birthday party; it was when I did some work with Billy Squier, so we're talking '83 or '84, and oh my God: tequila shots. I did eight and I don't drink and you know that even three would get someone really high, so of course I spent the rest of the night in the bathroom. It was terrible and I had such a wonderful girl to spend that night with me. We'd just started dating and I completely screwed that up.

CHIP Z'NUFF: That's a toughie because if you've been doing little extra-curricular activities like pills, blow and whatever the case of alcohol, it's always going to shorten the run. Nowadays we have Cialis and Viagra and Chinese Arithmetic, so there are things that will help you. I think your best bet is to just try and go into that situation without being inebriated and you'll have a chance. Those pills – not from personal experience but from what I've been told – seem to give you a little bit of confidence too. So if you're having a problem where you can get a rig but can't hold it, those certain pills can help you. You can drop that and it'll give you confidence, then sooner or later you won't have to use those pills any more, because you'll build up an immune system anyway.

COURTNEY TAYLOR-TAYLOR: Maybe sometimes you just can't after a big night. I have done the 'keep it together, don't drink too much' thing. 'Don't do too many drugs so you…' Or be 16 years old, that's the other way, although it lasted until about 28 with me. I could be just hurling, vomiting in the bathroom at a friend's party, and on the rare occasion that some girl came in to hold my hair out of the toilet or whatever and seduce me while I was throwing up, I lasted a long, long time. But nowadays if I'm a messy, shitty drunk throwing up, it ain't going to happen.

DANKO JONES: I don't drink and I don't really partake in too much of that stuff, so I'm pretty much ready to go. I've gone out with an alcoholic – full-blown. It's not a fucking party. It sucks if the other person's there and you can't do anything.

DOUG ROBB: Don't drink too much; that's pretty simple right? You get the whiskey dick. And don't over-think anything. If you're drunk or something like that and you're afraid you're not going to be able to get hard, then you're not going to get hard. You have to just kind of stay in the moment. Just enjoy what you're doing and everything will work out naturally, but if you start to freak out about it, that ain't going to help.

EVAN SEINFELD: Number one: cocaine is not an aphrodisiac. It's really cool when some girl is snorting it off your dick; it makes people think it is. For some reason, people have it in their mind that it's a sex drug, but it's actually an anti-erection drug. When I used to do cocaine I fucked for hours with a half-erect penis and would think I was a real stud because I couldn't cum, but the girls couldn't feel it either, so... I've been sober from drugs and alcohol for 20 years. I think there are some things like wine and champagne, a drink or two, that are good to loosen up certain inhibitions. I think if there wasn't Xanax, there might not be anal sex. I miss the good old days of Quaaludes and I think that there's a place and time for certain drugs. I'm not a fan of things like Ecstasy, invented drugs like that that you feel the long-term effects really negatively. There are really good natural male enhancement formulas that are more psychological than anything. Something simple like Horny Goat Weed can make a man feel a little edge and like he's going to be a stud because the male erection is completely in the mind. As a guy who's performed in over 200 videos on camera with 99.9% perfect success rate, it's like, it's in your head guys.

HANDSOME DICK MANITOBA: The only couple of times I ever had a hard time with an erection was after a tremendous night of being stoned, while I was very stoned. All I can tell you from a guy who hasn't had a drink or a drug in 25 years... I've had no erection problems in 25 years, so my attitude is get stoned or get laid. I don't think the two mix well.

JAMES KOTTAK: I've never had that problem.

JESSE HUGHES: Oh, getting turned on by girls. That works for me.

JIMMY ASHHURST: Try not to overdo it on the blow. Pretty much anything else should keep you going... although if you're that drunk, maybe a judicious amount of cocaine will help you out. But if you get that drunk, chances are you'll do too much blow anyway. I've found el naturale is the way to go for keeping the pecker up. I of course found that out way too late.

LEMMY: Don't have a big night. If you're that desperate for a fuck, don't drink. But then again you see, it's individual too. Some people don't seem to have a problem. Other people can't get it up no matter, even if they hit it with a stick; maybe they should tie it to the stick.

NICKE BORG: You have to plan. If you have the night out, or want to do whatever, or even if you're a fucking diehard drug addict, you still have to think of what's the most important thing – to do another line or get laid? Mostly I always use my friend's saying that I prefer the drugs better than the women, which is sometimes true depending on… But once you start to get professional, you can learn to handle it.

ROB PATTERSON: Well, I'm sober so I don't have this problem any more.

TOBY RAND: One way to cure that is a lot of visual stimulation – that always helps. I honestly think that it takes time and visual stimulation. If the lights are out and you're fucking hammered, your mind's not there. You need to be able to see what you're looking at 'cause you're too pissed to actually focus. You need to be able to focus and know what you're getting yourself into, 'cause then it'll take charge no matter what.

VAZQUEZ: Basically I'm a little different from most people as I don't really drink that much at all. And I don't do any drugs. I'm very different from whatever the stereotype is. I've got a whole different ball game and I never have that problem where I'm like, 'Oh fuck!'

Is sex generally better under the influence of drugs or alcohol?

ACEY SLADE: Nah, I don't think so. I think it can be more fun if your partner is fucked up because they might be a bit more agreeable to a third input or something, but for the most part drugs and alcohol are desensitising things that make you feel less.

ALLISON ROBERTSON: No, I don't think so at all. I think that it can be, but I think it also sucks if one of you is drunk or on drugs and the other one isn't. That isn't always so great. If both of you are, maybe, but I've seen it turn pretty disastrous if everybody's wasted.

BLASKO: I don't think it's better or worse. Let's put it this way: I think it's a fun thing to do if you're partying with someone equally as much. But if someone's partying and you're not, or if you're partying and someone else is not, then it's not as much fun that way. If both people are partying, then it's more fun.

BRENT MUSCAT: No, I don't think so; not at all. I think it's better when you're totally sober and you're all there. When you're having sex you have all the hormones and everything is raging through your body, so you should enjoy the feeling that you're getting. If you're numb with alcohol or on drugs, you're just not going to feel it as much.

CHIP Z'NUFF: No it's not. I don't think it is at all. I've tried them both ways. No. I think it's better with a little bit of pot and maybe a little glass of wine or something – that's fine. You're not inebriated then. You haven't stepped over the foul line. The other stuff is what gets you because first of all you don't get a rig and then you lose your sexual integrity and that's embarrassing. Then of course it kills the whole vibe. So my recommendation is a little wine, a little puffy-poo, and then attack.

COURTNEY TAYLOR-TAYLOR: No, I have no correlation between drugs, alcohol, sobriety and the relative quality of sex and the explosive intensity of it. There's no relationship that I can tell whatsoever.

DANKO JONES: With alcohol, I've noticed with people there's a point where it's good. It can actually start things because inhibitions are lowered and you can really have some good times, but from what I've observed in my experiences it's a window that opens and closes very quickly. Pretty soon the person is ready to pass out so inebriated that sex is impossible, no matter how much they say they want it. It's just impossible, so you just put them to bed.

I DEFINITELY THINK THAT UNDER THE INFLUENCE OF ALCOHOL YOU TEND TO BE MORE AGGRESSIVE AND LESS INHIBITED.

DOUG ROBB: I don't know if it's necessarily better. It's not like it feels different but your mind-set is a little different. I definitely think that under the influence of alcohol you tend to be more aggressive and less inhibited. So for those of you who are a little timid and want to open up a little bit, I would say give it a shot.

HANDSOME DICK MANITOBA: No, nothing is.

JAMES KOTTAK: You think it's better but it's actually better without either. It's an illusion.

JESSE HUGHES: Sometimes it is and like the Blue Diamond Viagra you can become Blue Diamond Phillips and star in any movie. That kind of shit – that's a tough question to answer isn't it?

JIMMY ASHHURST: It can be more intense. I wouldn't say better... at least you may think it was; you may think that you're performing like a fucking gladiator but chances are you're fucking not. It's taken me years and years of trying to find the right concoction of chemicals and alcohol to do it right and it's something you find out with time: the magic concoction is what you were pretty much born with.

LEMMY: It's great on acid; I'll tell you that. It's like your brain exploded. It's great fun but you couldn't do it all the time.

NICKE BORG: Sometimes you're under the impression that it's better because you're sometimes a bit more wild in your head, but I would say when you're a bit hungover the morning after is when it is best.

ROB PATTERSON: No, no, no, no, no! 100,000,000% better sober!

TOBY RAND: In the last year – yes. It has been a lot of fun. When it comes to the actual feeling of sex, it's better when you're sober, but the fun of sex is better when you're drunk because if you're with a different partner on a different night, all inhibitions are gone. It's like you've known them for ages and you just have more fun.

VAZQUEZ: I would definitely say no. I like to be fully aware and fully responsible for myself when I'm making bad decisions.

How do you know when someone is too intoxicated to have sex with?

ACEY SLADE: I guess if they still think you're the tour manager.

ADDE: I'm always more drunk, so I don't know.

ALLISON ROBERTSON: When they seem like they're just doing the same thing and it's not going anywhere… and they smell like whiskey.

ANDREW W.K.: I guess if they are puking. That's the most disgusting thing. And just that grogginess that comes over somebody where their body isn't working the right way. If they stink of liquor too; if there's so much liquor coming out of their system through their pores, chances are it's going to start coming out of their other openings.

BLASKO: I suppose whenever they throw up on you.

BRENT MUSCAT: When they're passed out and not responding. When they've got their eyes closed and you say, 'Hey honey!' and they don't talk and they're sleeping. I would say that's a good sign that you should leave them alone.

BRUCE KULICK: That's a turn-off for me too. On occasion, obviously there's been a girl or two that have… First of all, I wouldn't really date a woman who is like that because that's just a real turn-off to me. It's not the way I roll and also I don't really want to be with somebody that's all fucked up; I just don't. I'm not going to enjoy myself. I know that some guys are like, 'Oh this is going to be easy', but for me it's again about that connection and feeling that this person is cool to be around. If they're all screwed up, how are they cool to be around? I'm going to wind up baby-sitting them, or like in the movie *Almost Famous* calling the police and getting an ambulance for them because they overdosed. I remember this one story and it was kind of like one of my biggest *Penthouse* moments. I was touring in like 1975 and I'm in Madison, Wisconsin and I remember after playing this club that these two really pretty college girls picked me up and took me back to their place. They had a split-level townhouse. It was beautiful and I remember they were all into having me there and I thought, 'Oh this is *Penthouse* letters, here we go!' The two of them were kissing on the couch in front of me and I was like, 'Oh, this is unbelievable!' I was getting so excited about it but they were busy doing Quaaludes – Quaaludes being muscle relaxants, downers. Then one of them – actually it was the one I was more attracted to – got kind of sick. All of a sudden they didn't feel good. All of a sudden it was like that's it; she passed out and went to the bathroom and that was that. I still had fun with the other girl who could maybe handle her drugs, but the fantasy of having them both just went out the sky. But at that time in my life, anything and everything was exciting to me, but I'm still proud I got to see them kissing like that in front of me; that was fun. But it goes to show that, first of all, if you're doing a lot of drugs and drinking and then getting yourself in a sexual situation, you're not going to have the best sex. Neither of you will; it's bullshit. It's like you're escaping from something. Sex should be enjoying something and why would you want to be all screwed up for it?

CHIP Z'NUFF: Well you can't tell a guy that because if a guy meets trim and she's jacked-up out of her mind, it's not going to stop him. It's not a deterrent. He thinks it's going to be easier to close that deal. However it's not fun at all. You know right away by their behaviour, how they talk, how they carry themselves. That's a red flag immediately. Usually when guys are with girls who are inebriated, they're inebriated too, so it's masked a little bit and you can't really read it. But if you're seeing silly little things and she's acting stupid and throwing up, get away from her. Or if she's a friend of yours, take her home and drop her off.

COURTNEY TAYLOR-TAYLOR: When they basically can't be the aggressor.

DANKO JONES: It just sucks. The intent is there, the desire is there, but the execution of it just sucks and I'd just rather pass. Not wanting to be crass but just fucking jerk off and forget about it.

DOUG ROBB: You can just tell. It's all in the body language. Usually, if you're intoxicated with somebody and you guys are both going, if you feel like you're pulling way ahead in your aggressiveness or somebody's not responding as you thought, you should maybe take a step back and think, 'This is too messed up.' You want to keep it equal; you guys want to be equally intoxicated.

EVAN SEINFELD: Usually the vomiting is a pretty good sign; cleaning vomit off your penis. I'm really turned off by drunk women, so it's not something I encounter very much. But ladies – not cute.

GINGER: With tolerance levels differing, there is no set level of inebriation to watch out for. I'd say that for a new partner, if you've had more than a bottle of wine together it's not going to be as memorable as it could or should be.

HANDSOME DICK MANITOBA: Probably when they say, 'What's your name again?'

JAMES KOTTAK: When you're cleaning the puke off the pillow.

JESSE HUGHES: When they keep calling you Larry.

JIMMY ASHHURST: If there's vomit involved, that's usually the point. Or if their head's going around like in *The Exorcist*, you know that they're having the dreaded bed-spins and that's pretty much the point of no return.

JOEL O'KEEFFE: When she vomits heaps or passes out; it's best to let a sleeping dog lie.

LEMMY: When she throws up on you usually, and if she wants it, you're going to be a little put off by it.

NICKE BORG: When they start to talk about 7" vinyls while you are eating them.

ROB PATTERSON: Well, with my girlfriend, never.

TOBY RAND: When they are leaning over a bathroom bowl, throwing up saying, 'Don't worry, I'll be fine.' That's how I know they're too intoxicated. There's the old cliché that when they're throwing up they clench tight and it feels better, but that's when I know the line's been drawn in the sand mate.

VAZQUEZ: If you're looking at her and you're like, 'Damn, I think this girl's going to puke in my fucking bed', then that's when you know. To me it's not sexy. It's like, 'You know what, go home and be somebody else's problem. I don't want to baby-sit you. I'm not going to put my dick in you either.'

Any tips for the use of Viagra?

ACEY SLADE: Never had to use it. There are some nutritional things I've tried that are more like stimulants, not so much for getting an erection. There's this stuff called Vivaxl, which is an all-natural effervescent. You put it in your drink and drink it, then like a half-hour later your face just feels really flush; that's pretty cool.

ANDREW W.K.: I've never used it and I've heard it's amazing and I would really like to use it. It would just be a fun drug experience. I'm a younger man still and I've not gone down the road of Viagra, but I've had friends who have been heavy into cocaine for example (another thing that I've not really done a lot of) and that supposedly makes it very hard sometimes to be aroused, even more than alcohol. So they have this whole routine; these guys who are really into it. I definitely live vicariously through a lot of my friends who live these lives like out of a movie where they move to New York, they have a cool job, they live downtown, they go out every night (because you can in New York) and drink until four or five in the morning, do a bunch of cocaine with some girl that they pick up who likes the idea of doing lots of cocaine and gets a bunch for free, then take Viagra and have sex. The whole theme of the drug experience isn't the sex; it's about getting this high, the thrill of the pursuit, to all the drinking that makes it so much fun, to doing cocaine where you really truly are taking it into euphoric places and then crowning it off with the most euphoric of all, which was the sex. That just sounded really amazing to me, really great, but I've never done that. Something also about Viagra sounds a little scary because they say that... my friend who took it who also never has needed it but he took it for a drug experience; he's much older than I am and has a wife and he said that it was a little crazy because after five hours, it's not only that you're still aroused but you're mentally aroused too. You want to still have sex. That sounds like a good thing if you can set aside a whole day; take Viagra and even if you're by yourself, have a great time.

BLASKO: I haven't had to use it. I do know people that don't really have an issue but use it as a recreational sort of thing. You hear stories about dudes knocking over lamps and punching holes in walls accidentally just because they've got no control over it!

BRENT MUSCAT: I would not recommend it to someone. I think some people use it recreationally. Guys use it sometimes when they don't really need it. They can get hard and stuff but I think they think maybe it'll make it even harder or maybe more fun. I just don't think they should really use it unless they really need it, because I think you could become dependent on it somewhat. I heard that; I don't know. I tried it I think one time, probably like eight years ago and it works; I got hard, but I don't know how much different it was because I could get hard anyway. But I would tell guys that if they're having trouble, definitely go for it. If it works for all the men who are having some problems, I think it's a great invention.

CHIP Z'NUFF: Yeah, don't take the whole pill at one time like a dumb-dumb without drinking any water. Start off with a quarter or half a pill and drink a couple of bottles of water, then about an hour or two hours later you'll be ready to go. Be careful: it's not for everybody either. Anybody who's had heart conditions or problems with their blood should consult a physician before taking any kind of medication like that. For sure no alcohol and Viagra, although in Hollywood there are huge parties all the time and there's blow and Viagra passed out to everybody. It's like the best thing to do out there at these parties with some people – I won't mention their names because I don't want to hurt them. I don't recommend it. I don't think it's a good idea. I think you should be semi-together before you try any of that stuff.

START OFF WITH A QUARTER OR HALF A PILL AND DRINK A COUPLE OF BOTTLES OF WATER, THEN ABOUT AN HOUR OR TWO HOURS LATER YOU'LL BE READY TO GO.

COURTNEY TAYLOR-TAYLOR: Somebody gave me half-a-one one day and said, 'Dude, this going to be fun' and I slipped it into my phone book and I think I've lost it. A year later we were looking for it.

DANKO JONES: I've never tried it. Friends of mine have tried it and they've described the experience to me. It sounds wild man! When I heard, I was thinking, 'Man, maybe I should try some. It sounds wild!' But then it can have some serious side effects if you're young. So I'd rather not.

EVAN SEINFELD: If you're worried about having an erection, you're worried. If you need self-confidence, if that means taking a pill or popping a Viagra or a Cialis, do what you've got to do. I'm not a fan of those drugs; they have a lot of side effects. With the amount of sex my wife and I have, if I took those things I'd be addicted to them. The bottom line for me personally is that if you're not turning me on enough for me to be hard enough to cut diamonds…

HANDSOME DICK MANITOBA: I haven't used it yet. A lot of my friends tell me they've used it. I wouldn't be against using it; I'm not one of those people that's too proud in life to ask for help, but I haven't used it yet. I'll let you know for when you do the updated version of the book.

JAMES KOTTAK: Never tried it; don't need it.

JESSE HUGHES: Yeah, try not to if you don't have to and if you have an erection lasting four hours or longer that's talking to you, you're on acid.

JIMMY ASHHURST: Never tried it; haven't had to. I'm saving that for when my medical benefits kick in.

LEMMY: Well you take it or you don't; it's up to you. I wouldn't take it unless you need to because it's bad for your heart.

NICKE BORG: I've never used it dude. Seriously, I never felt that way to even try it. People can be like, 'Dude, I fucked for like three days' and I'm like, 'Jesus Christ! I'd fucking kill myself. Fuck for three days in a row?' And they're like, 'Yeah man, it was awesome.' Well, 'It couldn't have been awesome dude. The poor girl, shit!' I guess it's a good thing; I mean if people do have a problem, but if there's no problem, why?

ROB PATTERSON: Yeah, don't use it, unless you have to!

TOBY RAND: On my recent trip to Iceland I met a large security guy who said you should try one of these pills and he pulled out a bag of about a hundred blue pills. I said, 'What are they for?' and he goes, 'Trust me, with the girl you are with, you'll have a great time.' So my tip is never take one of those blue pills in a place like Iceland 'cause it's daylight the whole time and people can see your hard-on.

VAZQUEZ: I've never tried it; maybe I should because like, who knows? It might be really fucking crazy. I only get one bullet in the gun though and I can make it count. I can definitely make it count. My Dad tried it and he said, 'Oh man, it's fucking great!'

Is there a killer cocktail that can help secure a partner?

ACEY SLADE: That's where I've got to go back to my rock'n'roll and Jack 'n' Coke. Nothing is more rock'n'roll or more to the point than Jack 'n' Coke. I think it's a pretty surefire thing if you ask a girl, 'Hey, can I buy you a Jack 'n' Coke?' and she accepts. You're like 70% there.

ADDE: Probably a Long Island [Iced Tea] at the Rainbow Bar & Grill in Los Angeles. Leave out the Coke.

ALLISON ROBERTSON: Roofies [Rohypnol] always works. Ha! It's not good. Personally, I think that wine is not that great for feeling sexy. It always makes me feel angry and gets me into arguments with people. I would always say no about wine – not that that was the question, it was what you would drink. I think something that gets people more relaxed and in the mood and not really tense, so it would have to be something like a Margarita, tequila or something, although that can lead to barfing and that's never sexy. I think if you just have one or two, that's the key with any alcohol and having sex or anything romantic.

ANDREW W.K.: I always like Long Island Iced Tea because it's really fun to order. Every place kind of makes it different. You'll always be completely drunk after one; I mean, for me at least. Girls tend to like sweeter drinks from what I'm told.

BLASKO: If you're with somebody and you've got your eye on them and maybe striking up a conversation, you could always go for this one: you could say, 'Hey, can I buy you a drink but I'm going to pick what it is?' 'Sure, what's it going to be?' 'It's called the Flaming Jackass.' It's a shot of tequila with a teeny bit of orange juice on top and a bunch of Tabasco sauce on top of that in a salt-rimmed shot glass. Any time that you say, 'Hey, I'm going to get you a Flaming Jackass' I'm sure she'll get a chuckle out of that, and then the shot itself is pretty gnarly, so that's a good way to break the ice.

BRUCE KULICK: Because I'm not a big alcohol person, I wouldn't know. My only relation to that question is that I do understand that's a bit of an ice-breaker, to just offer somebody a drink, but it's up to them. I know which drinks are more potent than others, but everybody holds their liquor differently. I think those Appletini things – Apple Martinis, the real sweet ones – you can have two of those and the girl can be pretty looped. They're fun drinks because they're sweet and everything.

CHIP Z'NUFF: I hear that Jägermeister is very good at undressing. Other stuff I wouldn't really know about to be honest with you because I've never used those kind of tricks. I don't have personal experience with those things because I never do them.

COURTNEY TAYLOR-TAYLOR: I guess it depends. First instincts would be whatever they want, 'Let me buy you a drink. What are you drinking?' A fun thing to do is buy them a Scotch, just because it's classy and they'll try to drink some of it, then you can say, 'OK let's get something else.' Then you get them something else, you can finish their Scotch and they can have whatever they want, and you've quickly got a drink-and-a-half in them to see if you're getting anywhere. You've extended the length of your option to buy without having to finish your drink and then go, 'Another?'

DANKO JONES: It's not my style, I don't do that stuff. I'll buy someone a drink, but not in the hopes of getting them inebriated or lowering inhibitions. I don't roll like that. I really like to just make sure that the girl is into me because of me.

DOUG ROBB: I would say Cherry Coke; that's like my favourite drink. So if they ask why you ordered them a Cherry Coke you can at least say it's your favourite drink. It's probably the first Cherry Coke any guy has ever sent over to them.

EVAN SEINFELD: If chemical date-rape is your thing, for sure Jägermeister is probably the quickest path into her pants – albeit it's liquor. That's what to get if you don't want her to remember it.

GINGER: Tequila usually works wonders on a girl's inhibition, but no more than a shot or two. Exhibitionism in the wrong hands can be very ugly.

HANDSOME DICK MANITOBA: I was going to say tequila but that doesn't necessarily make people more sexual, it just makes them crazy. If a girl has a drink or two, that's one thing, but if a girl basically lives in bars and just drinks and drink and drinks, it's more of a warning sign. And I think it's the same for guys; I don't think it's just a girl thing. As a bar owner, the first thing I do if a guy says I want to buy that girl a drink is I always ask the girl if that's OK. It's old-fashioned but I don't want the girl to be uncomfortable. I always say, 'This gentleman would like to buy you a drink' because if you just hand it to the girl, some girls want the opportunity to smile and say, 'No, thank you.' I think it should be up to the girl to accept the drink or not. That's the way I like to run it. Basically, if a guy wants to buy a girl a drink, you go, 'I'd like to buy that lady a drink, whatever she wants.' Ladies first and whatever she wants.

JAMES KOTTAK: Long Island Iced Tea works every time.

JESSE HUGHES: You've got to be slick, so here's your first opportunity. A pick-up line doesn't have to be a phrase; a pick-up line can simply be being aware of something enough to see that that girl's drinking Cosmopolitans, so you have one slid down to her right as she finishes her last one. You be all cool, wait for her to look at you and smile.

JIMMY ASHHURST: Jägermeister, for sure. They call that the Panty Remover.

JOEL O'KEEFFE: Well, depending if they're already drunk or not, anything with fancy shit on it like curly straws, strawberries, cherries, umbrellas, mini swords or other stuff that has nothing to do with the actual drink usually works. When I'm buying a cocktail for a girl and she's not near me, I just ask the bartender to make whatever is the current most popular female cocktail and to chuck some fancy shit on it; works a treat!

LEMMY: I don't know. I've never bought cocktails really. It's just like down in the bars we frequent, I don't really go for the high-class John Collins or Singapore Sling stuff. If a chick wants one I'll by it for her, you know what I mean? I don't know. Probably eight vodkas because I suppose with chicks…

NICKE BORG: Just some really, really, really good quality red wine. It's great! Not too many glasses – a few.

ROB PATTERSON: I have no idea. Ha!

TOBY RAND: A Mojito given to me by my local watering hole The Vineyard, because it has extra, extra, extra alcohol in it.

VAZQUEZ: Whatever is free in the dressing room, that's what I'm offering. I'm not spending my fucking money on some woman, man. It's like, 'Oh Bud Light, well here you go honey! Let's get the romance started.'

ENLARGEMENTS & EXTENSIONS

"YOU'RE NEVER GOING TO MISTAKE REAL TITS FOR FAKE ONES BUT YOU CAN MISTAKE FAKE ONES FOR REAL ONES"

Are natural or enhanced breasts better?

ACEY SLADE: As long as they do the research and don't have any scars (that can be a buzz kill) by going through the armpit. I would definitely not suggest going through the underneath of the breast. But in a way, believe it or not, that kind of comes back to the personality thing: if a girl is secure, then a girl that doesn't have a large chest with a white tank-top on a hot summer day, I'll take that any day over D-cup fake boobs.

ADDE: I love small breasts. If they look really flat, I love it.

ALLISON ROBERTSON: I personally think that natural is better. I have friends that have enhanced and I think that works for them too, but I think that a lot of people who've had things done to their bodies actually wish they could go back to what they had before. That's kind of why I think natural can always be better because you can't go back once you've changed it, but if you keep it natural, you always have that option for later in life. Once you have implants and you get rid of them, you can't get rid of them without having a really weird, messed-up, loose skin situation. So personally, I'm a fan of natural.

ANDREW W.K.: Well, I have always preferred natural and I've never been able to fully grasp the appeal of implants. I understand them in theory. I've had friends who specifically like implants and don't like natural breasts. One friend in particular, this really amazing guy from Florida, who was just really hardcore into strippers and would make pilgrimages to Amsterdam once a month and just go crazy. He said, 'Andrew, I can tell you don't like implants but let me tell you what I like: I want them to look like two grapefruits cut in half, stuck up under there, rock hard, skin shining it's so tight, way far apart.' He specifically liked what some people would consider a badly done implant look. I really tried to relate to it, but I wasn't able to. I've seen implants that were very, very well done, but still it didn't look quite as good to me as a natural breast. The main thing is the psychology involved. The psychology of the woman who wanted to alter herself is very specific to the psychology of a woman who developed in a certain way and couldn't do anything about it. I admire and respect anyone that does plastic surgery. I think it's totally fine, but it comes from a certain head space of what you're trying to accomplish and I don't think it's specifically even a turn-off. I think someone changing the way they look to an idea that they have in mind is very exciting, artistic and very creative, but it means something when it comes to a sexual relationship. It has implications that I haven't felt arousing, whereas I've felt it very arousing to imagine a girl developing on her own and if she becomes extraordinarily well-developed, just the odds of that happening, the miraculous qualities of that happening, what her mind-set would be at having to watch her body develop, having to deal with the body that she has, how men and women react to her body, all those things to me are really exciting when it comes to someone being natural. It's the winning the lottery aspect where you just can't believe that this happened naturally that makes it so exciting.

BLASKO: Ah, enhanced.

BRUCE KULICK: Well, I have to admit that when you're young, it's real easy for the girls to have natural breasts that look amazing. Then that same girl you met when she was 20 that had a huge rack, if you meet them when they're 40, you'd run for the hills. The girls that had some breast enhancement – a boob job – didn't matter if they got them when they were 20 or 30, usually by 40 they're still looking pretty good, especially if they used a good doctor of course. So I can't say I have an issue with getting boob jobs. I think it's brilliant for girls; it balances out… I've met a lot of really pretty girls in my life that were not genetically blessed with a good rack and I think them buying it is fine. Even though it doesn't necessarily feel as natural, certainly when they're older, at least they've got some height as opposed to these things just hanging down to their toes.

CHIP Z'NUFF: There's something to be said about enhanced. As soon as you touch them you get a rig because they're so hard and firm and perfect. But I would prefer natural because you know that she's a natural person and she's not insecure about her looks. I prefer natural, absolutely. But like I said, there's something to be said for the enhanced. When you touch them, something happens.

I'VE SEEN IMPLANTS THAT WERE VERY, VERY WELL DONE, BUT STILL IT DIDN'T LOOK QUITE AS GOOD TO ME AS A NATURAL BREAST.

COURTNEY TAYLOR-TAYLOR: Natural, natural, everything natural.

DANKO JONES: Natural. Natural, all the way.

DOUG ROBB: I like natural breasts better, but I do like 'some' breasts. If you have absolutely no breasts, I wouldn't be against enhancements, as long as it's subtle. I don't want you to be flat-chested on Monday, then on Tuesday have the biggest rack. I think when you're obviously enhanced, it's kind of cool and fun to look at and go, 'Hey that girl's got big tits', but it's like wishing they were real.

EVAN SEINFELD: Good breast implants look perfect and last forever. I would say 5% of the women in the world are blessed with perfect natural tits that will stand the test of time and not succumb to gravity. So I think that young girls should enjoy their young, natural breasts while they can. I'm a big fan of quality breast implants.

HANDSOME DICK MANITOBA: Natural. As far as aesthetics or touch and feel for me, I prefer natural. Even if they're saggy, I don't care because I think it's better than hard or balloony-looking. Sometimes it looks better aesthetically in clothes, but not feel.

JESSE HUGHES: Natural. Somehow they seem more desperate and horny.

JIMMY ASHHURST: Ooh, that's a tough one. There's something to be said for some of these enhancements that are going around these days, at least visually. But when you stand them on their head and they're exactly the same shape as when they were vertical, it can be a bit suspect. There are a lot of shitty jobs going on out there – I live in the capital of them – I can't even remember the last time I had anything to compare one to; it's got to that point here. Of course, there are still a handful of women who have been blessed from birth and if you come across one of those these days you're a lucky man.

JOEL O'KEEFFE: Love 'em both! They're both fun to play with and both comfortable to sleep on.

LEMMY: Oh I like the enhanced ones. I went through years and years of natural ones; most of them are pretty bad news. Gravity asserts itself. Terrible thing that gravity. Why couldn't we have a bit less and be light-headed all the time?

NICKE BORG: I think natural breasts are the best, of course. I don't think you should fuck around with your body. But if you do feel very strongly that something's wrong with your body and you want to do something about it – and you're not fucking overdoing it – fine. And also these days – I'm not a professional on this stuff – but there's a certain density to it. You don't want to squeeze a handball; you want to squeeze a couple of tits, right? So it depends. I would think that chicks shouldn't do that. I know a girl that has the smallest fucking tits ever basically, but they're just fucking awesome because they're on her and it would just be so fucking ridiculous if she would get a boob job. I'd be like, 'What have you done?' But I don't judge anyone if they want to do that; it's up to them.

ROB PATTERSON: No difference to me.

TOBY RAND: Natural just feels better, but that being said, it all depends on what type of natural breast it is because enhanced breasts are also good. Ha! I'm torn between the two! If a natural breast sits up and is full and great, then definitely natural.

VAZQUEZ: Honestly, I'm going to have to say natural. As much as I love big tits, nothing is stranger than putting your hand on an enhanced breast: the skin feels good, but then you can feel that bean bag inside there and it's fucking weird man.

How do you determine if breasts are real or fake?

ACEY SLADE: You turn them upside down. Truthfully though, if it was a really good surgeon, you won't really notice.

ADDE: That's kind of easy to see because it's not natural the way those silicone tits look.

BLASKO: For me it's easy to tell when the clothes are off. Sometimes you can be fooled in this day and age. But whenever you can get your hands on them, you can just kind of tell.

BRUCE KULICK: I love people-watching and I love women, so I can obviously size it up pretty easy. Now, I have been fooled before because if a younger girl has had it done, I wouldn't necessarily know unless I'm physically grabbing them. Once again, a younger girl can have breasts that are perky and up there, especially if they got the normal boob job, meaning not the porn star look.

CHIP Z'NUFF: Oh you know right away once you touch them if they're real or fake, instantly. You just tell by the elasticity of the skin, the whole look of it. You're not going to meet a woman in her thirties with super-hard rock tits and not know! Unless you don't have any experience, then maybe I'm mistaken and you won't know, but for the most part you can tell right away.

COURTNEY TAYLOR-TAYLOR: All breasts are real. If you can't tell they're enhanced, then they're not. For God's sake, you don't want that creepy feeling of, 'If I squeeze this too hard it's going to pop out. It's not her; it's not a person.' There's something about being a person that gets me going. Like, it's them. It's their fucking reaction to it. There's nothing hotter than a woman feeling hot, feeling like she's really, really beautiful. It's just awesome. It's the most spectacular thing for a man to witness or be a part of.

DANKO JONES: If they're fake, your hand bounces back. It's like rubber.

DOUG ROBB: I don't know – most fake ones are pretty obvious.

EVAN SEINFELD: I think if you have to really ask you're never going to know. But guys, if you're a layman, look for the scars around the areola, or look for the scars under where the breast hangs. Look for the scar in the armpit. Put the girl on all fours and look for the ripples on the sides if she's thin. And know the feeling of it; know the feeling of nurturing silicone. It doesn't really matter though. I think big tits are kind of like *The Matrix*: if it looks good and it feels good, don't question it – just go with it.

HANDSOME DICK MANITOBA: I think it's obvious. I'm a fan of *National Geographic*, what can I tell you?

JAMES KOTTAK: The bounce factor: there's that little bounce up and down when they walk; you can see it.

JESSE HUGHES: Ask. I always ask immediately.

JIMMY ASHHURST: Oh, just a simple honk. Ha! I can usually tell. If you can't tell by the first honk, then she's probably got something interesting going on and you might want to continue the investigation.

JOEL O'KEEFFE: It doesn't bother me if they're real or fake. The fake ones are usually harder, but modern science is constantly making it harder to tell.

LEMMY: Well you can usually tell, although sometimes you actually can't. You're never going to mistake real tits for fake ones but you can mistake fake ones for real ones. I live in L.A., which is the centre of breast enhancement. It's always a bit disappointing going abroad.

NICKE BORG: Well you either have to be unconscious or a retard to not determine that.

ROB PATTERSON: Come on…

TOBY RAND: Firstly I can tell by talking to the girl for probably 20 minutes. Secondly, I can feel the texture of the boob. I'm all about boobs as well.

What steps should a woman take if considering an augmentation/enlargement?

ACEY SLADE: She should look at as many other women's breasts as possible and even if they're not considering getting their boobs done, most women should look at other women's breasts. Really though, it's just like anything else: go find your friends who have good boob jobs, go to a strip bar and see girls who have good boob jobs, find out who's gone to what doctors and avoid bad ones accordingly.

ALLISON ROBERTSON: I think you should research, get whatever the safest implant situation would be, like whatever the leak factor is. To me that's frightening; maybe some girls don't care but that's pretty frightening to imagine leaks in there. Also, I think the more money you spend and the research you do on the doctor, the recommendations and all that, go to somebody that somebody else you know went to and had success. To me the worst thing you can do is try and get a cheap one and that's there forever. They move, they change, so I think you want to spend as much money up front to make sure it's a good one.

ANDREW W.K.: I don't know; it sounds like something you could never really fully prepare for. I was going to say wear some sort of prosthetic device or those gel pads that enhance your breast size and walk around, but of course that's just going to encourage you to go for it even sooner; why even wait? You'll be psyched; it'll be great. It's an intense operation on one hand, but on the other hand you're putting a lot of energy into a very specific place, into a very specific side of the world of appearances and it's OK if that's what gets you off and where you want to go. I guess I would try to prepare someone and just say really get your awareness up and really be aware of what you're doing. There are many things to spend our time on, there are many things we can spend our money on and put our passion into and if this is one of those things that you want to do, just be very aware of the implications.

BLASKO: Go to a strip bar, look at the girls dancing and choose the one whose tits you like. Then go and ask her where she got them.

BRENT MUSCAT: She should check out a lot of girls who have had them done and look at them. She should touch other girls' breasts that have had it done and talk to a lot of other women who have done it, because by checking out a lot she should see good jobs and bad jobs. She should probably find the right doctor by finding the good jobs and feeling them. By talking to other women, she can also find out about the complications and stuff to see if she really wants to do it, because I know it hurts and there could be adverse side effects. Then, if you have them, eventually you have to have them re-done, so there's not just one surgery involved; you're going to have to have them re-done eventually. So it's multiple surgeries and any time you go under the knife, there's always a danger of dying too, so it's a pretty serious thing I think people should consider.

BRUCE KULICK: I know girls that are attractive and they wanted to do it and they did go pretty large and that made them feel better. I don't always agree with that because they have to hide them if they want to take a business meeting, you see? So I like it when a girl has done it so it's just appropriate for their physique. If they want to be a porn girl or a stripper, fine; just go for it and do it as big as your back can handle it. Who cares? You're going to be a stripper or a porn girl anyway. But if you want to be a normal girl-next-door, don't go too big.

CHIP Z'NUFF: She'd better get a couple of opinions, that's for sure. Go to a few different doctors. My recommendation is don't get them too big. For a chick that's 5'7-5'9, no more than a C, and for a girl that's between 5' and 5'4, I'd stay with a B. It's going to suit your body better and it's not going to hurt you. You don't need all that stuff inside you. It's unhealthy. It's not natural. You weren't born with fake tits and fake rigs. But definitely go to a couple of different people and talk to a few different doctors and get a second or third opinion to make sure you're making the right decision, because it's really hard to turn around. All the girls I know that had those and they got them too big, they had to go back to their doctors to get a reduction and that's expensive and sometimes painful and it could be dangerous.

GO TO A STRIP BAR, LOOK AT THE GIRLS DANCING AND CHOOSE THE ONE WHOSE TITS YOU LIKE. THEN GO AND ASK HER WHERE SHE GOT THEM.

COURTNEY TAYLOR-TAYLOR: Move the fuck out of Hollywood.

DANKO JONES: She should look in the mirror and learn to love herself and everything she was born with. Just be happy and content, because the chances are that mirror has been warped and she's probably completely fine and could turn on a lot of men, more than she thinks.

DOUG ROBB: I would definitely say keep it tasteful. Consider your frame size; consider what it is that you want out of it. Do you want to be known as the girl with big fake tits, or do you want to have breasts that people can't tell if they're fake or not?

EVAN SEINFELD: I think she should see the work of the surgeon in person, and multiples. She can look at a photo album but she should ask to see the actual doctor's work. If the doctor can't produce, my thought is she should not walk, but run! It's the woman's right to choose.

HANDSOME DICK MANITOBA: I always tell women, 'Don't do it.' But anything to do with surgery, you should see the work done, talk to people who've had it. It just seems like nobody's ever happy with what they have. They always want curly hair if they have straight hair; straight hair if they have curly hair, and so on. But, I don't live inside of them and if it's going to make them happier...

JAMES KOTTAK: Move to LA.

JESSE HUGHES: She should take four steps back and not do it.

JIMMY ASHHURST: Spare no expense: you get what you pay for unfortunately.

LEMMY: Take another job I should think; save up. They're expensive now.

ROB PATTERSON: Call her doctor? Ha!

TOBY RAND: I love to see… not over-the-top-sized breasts. I love a good C to D size that's natural looking.

VAZQUEZ: I'd just tell her not to do it, unless she's like a fucking man – an A cup. But if it's like you've got some nice Bs, then just keep them because you're going to look stupid when you get all that shit done. I really don't like it man; maybe I'm crazy, but I don't like it.

When should a penis extension be considered?

ACEY SLADE: If he has to repeatedly say, 'It's in', I guess.

ADDE: Probably never – you should work on your fucking moves instead.

ALLISON ROBERTSON: I think if you're frightening girls with how small it is. I think guys know. I think that there's always a girl that belongs with the guy, so I think that everybody can find their match size-wise. I don't think just because you have a little wiener you have to have an extension. I think if you go through life and you just find girls are dropping like flies and running away, which I've known girls to do, me included. It's mean but it's kind of true. A lot of girls just know that they can't really handle that, so I think if it's really hard to find a partner or someone that doesn't care. To me, boob jobs and penis mods are really personal and it's more about yourself; if it makes you happy and that's what you want. I think it's lame to do anything for another person unless you're like married and they really, really, really want it. As far as other people in general, I've never been a fan of any of that stuff unless it's really for you.

ANDREW W.K.: The idea of that is one of the greatest ideas that clearly

has taken the male population of the world by storm. It's probably the most appealing concept in the world and I imagine there isn't any man, no matter how well-endowed or how small he may be, that hasn't thought about that idea. It's like flying; it's like being able to fly. I don't know why it's something that's so appealing, but we've heard that many times where women say it doesn't matter, it's how you use it, not what it is or how big it is or how small it is. I remember specifically that when girls have said they've been with someone too small, it didn't come down to the way it felt so much, it came down to the way that guy felt about his size, how he behaved and how he carried himself. I imagine it would be like someone who had issues with how tall they are. For a man, that's apparently a very intense head space. I've been very grateful for the way I've been made physically in every way, as much as I would be for just being able to walk or being able to hear and having my eyes work. I'm grateful in a very all-over way. I think it's a very specific fantasy for a man (and maybe for women too) and the phallus as it stands in the human psyche is a very elemental, primal thing. It takes up a lot of space I think in everybody's brain. A friend of mine says, 'All men think about dick. Gay men just think about it a lot more.' I thought that was probably right. The very nature of sexuality is all wrapped up in the idea of a dick going into a hole and when you have one of those dicks, it's a big part of your life. So wanting it to be even bigger seems to make perfect sense to me.

BLASKO: Never! I've read things about that and it's like it doesn't work

properly. It ends up being like a sausage in a tube sock or something. Like, it's all there but there seems to be some kind of issue… like, that seems kind of tricky to me dude – I wouldn't get anywhere near that.

BRENT MUSCAT: I guess if you have a deformity maybe, or if you have

an accident. I would never advise it unless you *really* need it. I wouldn't advise operating on the penis unless it's like an emergency.

CHIP Z'NUFF: If your little rig is two to three inches, maybe then an

extension might help you. I've got to be honest with you: if you were born like that, learn how to dine. If you dine, women love men that dine and then you can put that little baby rig inside of them and you'll tickle them for five seconds and you're done and you'll come off like a champion still.

DANKO JONES: I can't even think of that without cringing and grabbing my dick. I can't even think of someone going down there to do that… No! No, you shouldn't do that either.

EVAN SEINFELD: I didn't know they actually did that. But I think guys, when your female partner tells you that size doesn't matter, that means it really does. Because guess what? It does.

JESSE HUGHES: When you're hung like a horsee, instead of a horse.

JIMMY ASHHURST: Oh man, I don't know which sort of extensions are available now. I guess the surgical one and the Swedes have had those fucking contraptions like pumps and things – you can always get a good laugh out of seeing one of those. But I don't think an extension should ever be considered unless it's like… whatever the fuck you've got, work with it.

NICKE BORG: They say that size doesn't matter, which is complete bullshit. I don't know man; that's a hard question. I don't even know anybody that has asked me, 'Do you think I should get a penis extension?' Ha! I have no idea, but if there's something that really fucking bothers you, like you have the smallest fucking cock in the world… but dude, we're in the generation where we watch dwarves having sex with porn stars or whatever!

ROB PATTERSON: For me, never!

TOBY RAND: When you have a small penis.

Do you think partners prefer a circumcised penis or natural?

ACEY SLADE: I'm circumcised but I don't know. Most girls that I know, and granted a lot of them are Americans, think that the uncircumcised looks like an anteater and I can't imagine wanting to put an anteater in your mouth or any other part of your body, so I'd say circumcised.

ADDE: Probably circumcised, but I would like them to prefer natural because that's who I am.

ALLISON ROBERTSON: I've known a lot of girls who have a preference but I don't think it matters at all. I think they're both nice.

ANDREW W.K.: I think the girls I've been with have said circumcised. I am circumcised so I'm sure that had something to do with influencing their answer.

I think there's this idea with women that it's cleaner when you're circumcised but that just comes down to showering and bathing. I don't really think there's something inherently cleaner or not. I haven't talked a lot about that with girls.

BLASKO: I'm uncircumcised and I haven't had any complaints, so let's just leave it at that.

BRENT MUSCAT: I don't know; I wouldn't know about that. I'm circumcised, but I've had friends that are not circumcised too and I guess the only difference they tell me is they have to keep it a little cleaner. Sometimes there's an issue with cleanliness. I don't know. I guess if you're not circumcised there's more skin so maybe you're a little bit bigger.

BRENT MUSCAT: I'm circumcised; I'm Jewish. I was born and had the rabbi and the ceremony and the whole thing, OK? That's traditional in America anyway – usually they do the circumcision – but in certain countries it isn't. Like, when you watch foreign porn, you're like, 'What's that on that guy's dick?' You get what I mean? Being a New Yorker and an American, I don't know a lot of guys that aren't circumcised or don't know what their lovers would think if they weren't, so it's hard for me to comment on that. I know that when I have seen it in porn, it is always a little weird to me. 'What's going on there?' In certain countries, of course, that's more the norm and being circumcised is unusual, so it all depends on where you come from.

CHIP Z'NUFF: Most women I know don't want uncircumcised penises because a) it's not clean, and b) it looks scary to them. I recommend circumcised. When I had my little son I had him circumcised for sure and I think it's healthier that way too for the kids, from what I've been told through doctors.

COURTNEY TAYLOR-TAYLOR: Everyone in movies, girls gossiping in dialogue and shit, the cliché is circumcised.

DANKO JONES: I don't know, I never really thought about it. Oh fuck, I don't know.

DOUG ROBB: I would think circumcised but I don't know. I kind of figure that circumcised is cleaner, and clean is good.

EVAN SEINFELD: I hear from more and more women that circumcised is a non-negotiable, but there are women who are completely into the fetish of a fellow's foreskin – an unaltered self. I mean, you've got what you've got.
My friend Iggor got circumcised at age, I think, 28. I give him all kinds of respect for being like the fucking most hardcore dude ever, because that fucking takes guts! I think it's a personal preference thing. I think guys, there's no point in even asking a woman because you're not going to get your foreskin back if she's

like… and you probably don't have the balls like Iggor has to get cut. So if you're natural and she likes circumcised, well maybe it's time for a threesome with a guy who's different.

GINGER: I think anyone who dislikes your penis, cut or otherwise, is probably a very bad match.

HANDSOME DICK MANITOBA: I don't know. I've never heard anyone say, 'I wish you weren't circumcised.' I didn't have any choice in the situation.

JAMES KOTTAK: I couldn't even guess man.

JESSE HUGHES: It seems these days they want it big and somehow ethnic. Other than that, I don't know. I think when people want to get down they want it to be big.

JIMMY ASHHURST: I've never really asked anyone if they prefer the anteater but I, being circumcised, would hope that they'd prefer the circumcised version.

LEMMY: Well I've only ever had a natural one; I've never been circumcised. I don't recall ever having a rejection.

NICKE BORG: That comes back to what country you come from, or what kind of religion you have. In Sweden, at some time people did it, but mostly didn't. I think if you don't usually take a shower every day, maybe it's better to be circumcised. If you do have a shower every day, I don't know… It needs to be for a medical reason I think, otherwise it's fucking phoney.

ROB PATTERSON: Ewww.

TOBY RAND: It depends on where you go… different countries. For instance, in Australia circumcision is not that common I think – well within my circle of friends it's not that common, so I don't think anyone has a problem with it. But in America, some girls you might be with are not used to it. But in the end, I don't think it has anything to do with that, it's just how you use it.

VAZQUEZ: I've never even asked women that, man. Me, I'm circumcised, and I've had no complaints.

FETISHES & FANTASIES

"ONE OF THE STRANGEST FETISHES THAT I'VE ALWAYS MARVELLED AT IS WHEN GIRLS WANT ME TO PEE ON THEM"

What's the best way to make sexual fantasies come true?

ACEY SLADE: These things kind of go two ways: there's the sleazy side of it with the girls backstage and two girls alone with you is a box of chocolates; you just party. But it's been my experience that if I'm with someone I love, all the crazy shit goes out the window a little bit.

ADDE: Start a rock'n'roll band and just practise like fuck. Then just go out and play the world.

ALLISON ROBERTSON: I think if you're good enough friends first, to be able to talk about this stuff without it being awkward. I think it's a bad idea to tell a girl what to do, and maybe the same to a guy. I feel it's lame. If you have a fantasy, or a fetish or two, or anything like that where it's kind of customised, I think it's really lame to boss the other one around and tell them to do this or do that. I think it makes more sense to get to know each other a little better and maybe have one or two bad or awkward situations, and then find out what the other one likes and figure it out from there and customise it and make it more fun. To me, I don't like being ordered around and I also know I can be bossy in general, but I think it's a turn-off when either one is not comfortable trying to please the other one and is kind of afraid.

ANDREW W.K.: First decide if you really want them to because once you do it, it's no longer a fantasy. That's my thing. The fantasy is empowered by the fact that it's not real and, while that could seem like it's less thrilling than actually doing it, the control that one has with one's imagination is much more easily manipulated than the control someone can have over someone else in a 'real-life' encounter.

BRENT MUSCAT: I guess be open with your partner or partners. Being in a band is always good; being in a popular band was great for me as I got to do a lot of fun stuff. I guess one of the most fun things was having two girls in the back of the bus. Having two girls going down on me was awesome, but I don't know if I would have been able to do that if I wasn't in a band. I'm pretty lucky that I had my time on tour.

BRUCE KULICK: I don't know if you can force that. I know sometimes when I make plans like, 'Oh my girl is going to fly in; we're going to be in Vegas. This is going to be great. I've got a beautiful room' and you can think, 'Oh, look at that chair! We'll do it on that chair.' Then maybe on that trip there's a lot of other stuff that comes up, that's called life, and you're lucky to have sex at all, let alone on that chair with lingerie. Then the times where you don't make any preparations or anything, you have the sexiest night and have the greatest sex. I think it's really hard to premeditate any of it and I think there's something natural with life… it just has to happen how it's going to happen, as opposed to you making some plans. I just think the great nights happen by themselves.

CHIP Z'NUFF:
That's a loaded question. The best way would probably be to just go pursue it with all the vigour you have and give it your all, but that might find yourself starting a relationship in a way you're not used to and she's not used to and it's phoney; so maybe natural. You see somebody and it trips your trigger and you say hello and talk to them for a little bit. If it gets to the point where you're going to spend some quality time with them, don't be selfish. That's my recommendation. Do not be selfish. Do it for them and in the long run it'll work out for you.

COURTNEY TAYLOR-TAYLOR:
I'm not even sure that making them come true is a good idea in the first place.

DANKO JONES:
It's interesting: if you're with someone, like you have a partner, and you want to incorporate some of your fantasies in the relationship and they're pretty wild, be prepared to wait a long fucking time. On the other hand, one-night stands or relationships that aren't really relationships, they're like friendships where you fuck, I think you stand a better chance of making those fantasies come true.

DOUG ROBB:
To be open about them. I think if you're comfortable with somebody and have fantasies – because everybody does – just be open about it. Don't be ashamed about that part of your life or your body or your mind or whatever. You should just be like, 'My fantasy is this. Take it or leave it.' If you tell me you don't have fantasies, you're lying to me and to yourself.

EVAN SEINFELD:
I think, with your partner, it has a lot to do with real honesty and not being afraid to tell your partner what your fetish is and what your fantasies really are, because your partner may surprise you and grant you your fantasy. Me personally, I'm living them all out every day: I'm married to Tera Patrick so… as much as I can take all the fruit, my fetish and my fantasy is to have sex with the most beautiful woman in the world every night and I do. But if I didn't tell my wife, 'Hey, I'm a pervert and I want to shoot porn with all kinds of girls and have my own website, rockstarpimp.com – the world's only celebrity rock star porn site' she wouldn't know and I wouldn't have been able to work it out with her. What you keep as your secret may never come to life, so be fearless, gentlemen.

HANDSOME DICK MANITOBA:
If you've got a good partner, tell them. Just tell them. I don't think you should depend on other people to think about what you feel and what you want. We walk around 24 hours a day locked inside

these things you see in the mirror and then all of a sudden it's like, 'OK, I've had these fantasies for 18 hours and I want you to know what they are.' You don't have to lay it out like a novel – guide them, guide them. Tell them you like this, you like that. Guide them and if you have a good partner they will take the guide and run with it.

HAVING TWO GIRLS GOING DOWN ON ME WAS AWESOME, BUT I DON'T KNOW IF I WOULD HAVE BEEN ABLE TO DO THAT IF I WASN'T IN A BAND.

JAMES KOTTAK: Go for it!

JESSE HUGHES: Opposites attract but birds of a feather flock together, so it's best to go where one would go to indulge in such a fantasy. If you're looking for the S&M culture, the best place to find it is not on Sunday in a Baptist church.

JIMMY ASHHURST: Find a willing partner would be the first step and, if you've got the right one, then anything you can concoct should at least be worth a try.

LEMMY: Oh, well that depends entirely on the sexual fantasy. If it involves biting people with fake fangs or a baseball bat, I don't know. There are all kinds of weird fantasies. You've got to have a partner who is interested in the same thing, otherwise the fucking thing is a non-starter from day one, isn't it?

NICKE BORG: I think that sexual fantasies should stay sexual fantasies because usually when you try to make them happen for real, they're not as cool as they were in your fucking fantasies. Sometimes I guess they can also turn out to be a catastrophe, like, 'Oh my God! I thought you wanted me to fuck your sister.' 'Yeah in my fantasy.' 'But dude, she liked it.' So I think that fantasies should stay that way otherwise there wouldn't be sexual fantasies – that's the whole fucking thing about it.

ROB PATTERSON: Do them!

TOBY RAND: Just tell your partner what you want.

VAZQUEZ: I feel like I've done every fantasy that I've ever really wanted to do. Honestly, for me, so long as the woman is fucking getting off and having fun, I'm fucking happy. If she wants to wear a schoolgirl uniform and do that, that's fine with me.

What's the strangest fetish a partner has asked you to participate in?

ACEY SLADE: An orgy that had a lot of guys.

ADDE: Oh there are so many things… the most would be when she wanted me to piss on her, but that's not so bad actually; it's kind of crazy.

ALLISON ROBERTSON: I don't know; I think that I've had some pretty boring situations. I'm trying to think. I've known some people who liked their hair pulled really hard and I think that seems like something a girl would like, so to me I was like, 'Ooh, that's kind of weird for a guy to go there.' So there's that and some guys ask me to say certain things, but other than that I've never really been with anybody that's necessarily freaky. Sometimes it's the way they ask that can make it feel weird.

BRENT MUSCAT: One of my friends called me vanilla the other day. We played an adult film museum, or something like that, and on the outside it said, 'Catering to kink and vanilla.' I was like, 'What is this vanilla?' and he was like, 'You're vanilla.' So I was like, 'What does that mean?' and he said, 'You just kind of like straight sex' and I would say I am into just straight sex mostly. So, most of the people I've been with have been pretty vanilla as well. But some girl told me once that she was going to screw me in the ass with a strap-on dildo and I said, 'No way! Forget that. I'm not into that.'

CHIP Z'NUFF: For me, I'm a pretty old-fashioned guy. I know that girls have always tried to stick things in me, but I don't dig that at all. I don't dig that at all and I always stop that before it starts. It wrecks any kind of romance that would have been building up.

COURTNEY TAYLOR-TAYLOR: Nothing seems that weird to me. There are weird dudes out there but I'm not going to go there. I'm a traditional guy. Getting naked, getting turned on and getting off with someone really hot is good enough for me. I love that. You mean there's something that's supposed to be better? Really? You know, if something's better than that, you're crazy!

DANKO JONES: Oh, I want to say this to you but I can't man; I can't. I could stop at just a three-way, that's been asked before although it's never happened to me; it's always been bandied about. Somehow, for some reason, fate has stepped in and screwed it up, whether it's the weather, they can't make it, the train broke down, whatever it is.

DOUG ROBB: My sexual career must seem very boring because I can't think of any strange fetishes. Fuck, I don't know. I'm going to have to think about that one.

EVAN SEINFELD: I hear about all kinds of things because I'm in the industry. I hear about things like trampling, where guys wants girls to walk on them and like run over them in high heels and shit. One of the strangest fetishes that I've always marvelled at is when girls want me to pee on them. I'm always like, 'What's that really about? What's the psychological profile behind that? Did your Daddy do something to you, or your Mommy not hold you enough?'

HANDSOME DICK MANITOBA: I knew you were going to ask questions about weird things like this because I guess it makes for good reading, but really my whole life I've had none of that. It's always just been the basics. I haven't done anything weird with machines or dressing up or whatever. In terms of the totality of what's out there and what people do, I'm a very basic, bland sexual animal.

JESSE HUGHES: One night two girls tried to put shit on and fuck me with it and I will tell you right now, with the good Lord as my witness, I will never do such! They were big-ass, hot girls, but muscle-builder style girls (think Chyna from WWF), and that shit scared me. I was like, 'Woah!' She would not take no for an answer baby.

JIMMY ASHHURST: There's this group of people that like the stuffed animals; they like to actually be the stuffed animals: Furries or Furverts they're called; it's an animal transformation fetish. I ran into one of them and it's an odd bunch. They actually have like meetings and conventions and all that sort of thing, and they like to dress up in life-size furry costumes… so that was interesting. I'm sure you'd have to have the holes in strategic places.

LEMMY: Well it wasn't me; it was the singer of a band I used to be in that shall remain nameless. We all slept in the same room; four of us. He was in bed with this chick and she suddenly says, 'Piss on me!' He said, 'What?' He was from Bradford in the north of England and not very well versed. She said, 'Go on! Piss on me!' So our bass player pissed on her instead I think. That's strange isn't it, that one? And that foot thing I never understood; you want to suck somebody's toes? Not me! Fucking hell. I'm pretty conservative in a way. I don't like anal sex either. I figure if shit comes out of it, I'm not going into it either.

ROB PATTERSON: I can't answer that.

TOBY RAND: The strangest would have been to watch her take a shit. She didn't want me to eat it or anything, but she wanted me to watch. I thought that was pretty strange… it's not really one of my turn-ons.

VAZQUEZ: I had an ex who was into… she liked to be choked a little bit when we were fucking. In some strange way that was kind of fun.

How do you know when you have a fetish, or just really like something?

ACEY SLADE: I don't know. It's been brought to my attention that I have an Asian fetish, but I clearly deny that. I guess denial is the first sign of having a problem. On a more serious note, if it's causing problems within your life and it's something you have to lie about, then it's a problem.

ALLISON ROBERTSON: I think a fetish is something where you can't have sex or you can't really get turned on without something in particular, as opposed to just having regular sex where it's pretty run of the mill. I think if you have to have a certain part touched or touch someone else's certain part, or you have to say something or they have to say something, or you need your hair pulled otherwise you can't have sex or finish, to me that's a fetish, as opposed to something you just like.

ANDREW W.K.: Maybe when the idea of that thing arises at any time or place and it arouses you… anything that relates to it or when many of your thoughts seem to trace back to that one thing that is somehow removed from an actual person, an actual experience, or anything logical. When it becomes an illogical turn-on, I guess that's when it becomes a fetish.

BLASKO: Whenever they make a magazine for it. Whenever you're subscribing to *Amputees Monthly*, then you know that you've got a fetish.

BRENT MUSCAT: I think a fetish is something that you're obsessing over; I think that's when it could be considered a fetish. I guess some guys have a foot fetish. Some guys have a thing with cigarettes where they like to see the girl smoking a cigarette or doing something weird, but I guess it's when you're into another body part that's not normally considered for sex. Like an ear! If you want some girl to jack you off with her feet, I think that's a fetish.

BRUCE KULICK: In that category, I don't think I'm very extreme in one way or another. I think a guy that has a fetish like, 'You've got to leave your shoes on' or 'You've got to dress as a boy' or whatever it is, I guess if there's something where the only way you'll get off is if they do something that's not normal, then you've got a fetish. I don't think there's anything wrong with that, so long as you've got a partner that's willing to play the game with you. I'm pretty straight ahead, where I don't feel like I have anything that unusual. Sex is so personal and it's so unique with everybody and certainly there are enough people where the norm is not enough. We're all wired very different.

CHIP Z'NUFF: I've got a foot fetish. I love hoofs and I have since I was a little kid and I know that women love their hoofs kissed and touched and rubbed. That's something that seems to work with almost *all* women. You massage them and that gets the ball rolling instantly.

COURTNEY TAYLOR-TAYLOR: The difference between normal and not-normal? I have no fucking clue. I have no idea where that grey area begins and ends. Google it – that's how you find out, you Google it.

DANKO JONES: I guess when you obsess over it and you notice no one else does.

DOUG ROBB: I think if you really like something, then it's the icing on the cake. If you like having sex and if you get to do something certain or specific, it's even better. If it's a fetish, it's the entire cake.

EVAN SEINFELD: I think it has to do with the amount of feelings around it, you know. I think you would need a third party to help you figure that out and make a choice. So let's say a guy really likes women's feet in stockings and he's not sure if it's a problem or not, you need a third party to say, 'OK, sex with a beautiful girl, or rubbing her feet?' Like a questionnaire or a quiz. '$500 or the girl's feet?' So you can come up with a standardised test where the third party thinks what you should choose over this thing... but once again, fetish is about personal turn-on preferences. There's no right or wrong to them, so long as you're not breaking any laws or harming anyone in the process. Like, if I've got a fetish to have girls wear fishnet stockings, well if I want to buy those girls fishnets then who am I hurting? Once a guy has multiple memberships to specific websites or more than 10 DVDs of a certain genre, I think it's a fetish.

JAMES KOTTAK: If it's the tenth time, it's not a fetish any more; it's habit.

JESSE HUGHES: When you fetishize it. When it accompanies you; when you treat it like a precious in *Lord of the Rings*. I watched Mel Brooks' movies forever and I've always noticed there's a little S&M fetish in there and every time I've watched it I've always been like, 'How is that possibly... How could anyone actually be into this fucking shit?' And truly, just by fucking around with it and being attracted to the style I guess, I find myself now carrying with me a little leather Lone Ranger mask with studs on it and a half goon mask. Now I know, because I like it.

JIMMY ASHHURST: If you're talking about it with some friends and suddenly the room goes quiet, that would be an indication I believe.

LEMMY: When you do it by yourself. When you find yourself hanging in the wardrobe with a ball gagging your mouth.

NICKE BORG: I guess after you try it, otherwise you wouldn't know.

ROB PATTERSON: I don't have a 'line' between these things.

TOBY RAND: I think fetish is a really broad category because everyone has their own little idiosyncrasies that they love about sex and what they want to do. So how do you know? When someone tells you it's a fetish, otherwise to me, anything's a go.

VAZQUEZ: I think it becomes a fetish when you can't be with anyone that doesn't please that fetish. I love voluptuous women and maybe that's a fetish, but to me, it's not. That's just what I like. If I met some girl who was really cool who wasn't like totally voluptuous, then that's cool.

What is your best costume experience?

ACEY SLADE: Myself and another bandmate of mine were dressed up as Paul Stanley and Gene Simmons for a Halloween. It was funny because we both got these Kiss slippers that looked like the Kiss boots. This was early in a tour and we both hooked up with this one girl and, after she left, anytime we saw Kiss slippers it would become a joke.

ADDE: I never wear a suit, but I had sex one time with a girl on a toilet at a wedding while wearing a nice suit and I found it to be like, 'Wow, this is so cool. Just hang out my cock and wear a suit,' so probably that time.

ALLISON ROBERTSON: I wish! I think costumes are cool actually; I really do. I think dressing up and stuff is kind of neat. You know what's funny about that? I feel like most guys want girls to dress up and wear lingerie – that whole girl thing – and girls want that too I think. But what sucks is that there really isn't much for the guys to do on that end and I would actually really like for there to be some costumes in my future. I don't know what kind. A businessman would be kind of hot!

ANDREW W.K.: I don't think I've ever had a costume experience.

BLASKO: I think that the doctor and patient is always a good one.

BRENT MUSCAT: That was one thing I liked about Japan: a lot of the Japanese girls would dress up. Costume play they call it there. They'd dress up like nurses and stuff. That was always fun. When I went out touring, a lot of the girls would come to the shows dressed super-sexy, just barely wearing anything. I remember doing an in-store and two girls came in wearing bikinis; anything different like that was always fun. When we toured with David Lee Roth, I remember the very first show we did was in the summer down in Miami, Florida and it was the first time I ever saw girls come to a show in bikinis. I was like, 'Wow! This is awesome!' you know what I mean? That's fun.

CHIP Z'NUFF: I prefer the birthday suit. The revealing in the beginning is always exciting. However with stilettos and corsets that suck everything in and make you look more chiselled and perfect, as soon as you take the shoes off and everything comes off, you know it all changes. Any time you meet a woman and they look fine, you see them in the clubs and they've got the high heels on and nice pants or nice dress, a beautiful bra, a top, and as soon as you get home, you take all the accessories off and you just get the frumpy, stumpy, squashy, dumpy – that happens sometimes. Women are very good at bamboozling us in the beginning. I prefer the birthday suit.

COURTNEY TAYLOR-TAYLOR: I grew up in a very small, depressed city of about 300,000 people. There was nothing to do. We could get into bars when we were 19 (21 is the drinking age). There was just nothing to do, so on maybe two occasions me and maybe a friend, we'd just dress up in drag and go out and have some drinks. So you go to Good Will or Value Village and buy some size 13 pumps and maybe like a tube dress and just the funniest wig you can find and you just go out and hit on ladies. It's funny and it's really fun and it definitely gets the nookie going.

DOUG ROBB: One Halloween I was the Pope and my girl at the time was a naughty Catholic schoolgirl. I'm pretty sure after that, it was an interesting night.

JAMES KOTTAK: Zorro!

JESSE HUGHES: Now see, I love costumes! I've had many a wonderful costume experience. I got to have a couple of fantasies indulged: Roger Corman biker girl fantasies, and having three girls dress up in red and black pirate-striped shirts with leather and denim vests on and biker boots, and me dressed up. That shit's hot and you fucking know this!

LEMMY: A chick once met me at LAX (Los Angeles International Airport) with a long coat on and she opened it as I got off the plane and there was a red lace bikini underneath it. We didn't even get as far as the car.

NICKE BORG: This is maybe not my best but it's absolutely the weirdest one: it was a chick who was dressed up as a rat, with a tail and everything. It was in Berlin; many, many years ago I have to say. She was dressed like a rat with these zippers and shit. Costumes are fucking cool you know, but it depends on what kind of girl is wearing it. Be a cop, be a nurse, be whatever, man. Just do it like you really mean you want to be a nurse and nurse me, or be a cop and want to beat me, whatever. Don't try and be a rat and bite me though.

I'VE DRESSED IN DRAG A FEW TIMES. IT'S FUN, BUT I DON'T KNOW HOW WOMEN WALK IN THOSE HEELS!

ROB PATTERSON: I've dressed in drag a few times. It's fun, but I don't know how women walk in those heels!

TOBY RAND: When a girl in Los Angeles dressed up in red Lycra like in the movie *Roger Rabbit*, but the Lycra was breakable. It was like a thick Glad Wrap and you could peel it apart. That was an awesome costume.

VAZQUEZ: I've never really done that. My birthday is Halloween and I don't want to be bothered with costumes, so my excuse is, 'I'm the King of Halloween – I don't have to fucking do this. This is *my* day; you do what I want.'

What's a good way to begin exploring bondage?

ACEY SLADE: Gaffer tape – there's always some of that around.

JIMMY ASHHURST: From personal experience, I'd say having a mentor. I was fortunate at a very young age to have a person I much respected and a very unlikely partner, who shall remain nameless. They both demystified the practice of bondage to me. It was quite interesting and there are lessons that have stayed with me until this day.

LEMMY: Bondage? Tie one of you up I suppose.

ROB PATTERSON: Try it! You'll know what works and what scares you or your partner. Always have a 'safe' word!

TOBY RAND: By slapping the ass harder and harder each time and seeing how far you can go.

FOREPLAY & AROUSAL

"I THINK IMPATIENCE IS THE MARK OF AN IMMATURE SOUL; THE LONGER YOU CAN HANGOUT THE BETTER"

How much foreplay is optimum?

ACEY SLADE: I'm a big foreplay fan. Generally, I like to take care of a girl twice before the act itself if it's the first time I'm with someone.

ADDE: A lot of foreplay, because for me foreplay is like teasing each other with words; starting with a conversation and taking it from there. So a lot of foreplay for me is best.

ALLISON ROBERTSON: I don't think it really matters. I think some people can wait forever and other people start getting like they're going to explode. To me, everything is case sensitive and you have to feel out the other person and decide. But I don't like it when people rush in. I'm not really into like if somebody just jumps on top of you. I like a little bit of something before anyone's making out. I think almost all girls do, unless there's something wrong with them psychologically and they're doing it for another reason. I think that almost all girls like that and some guys do too, but not all of them. So I think it all depends. I think you can tell if somebody is definitely excited and doesn't need any more.

ANDREW W.K.: Foreplay can be an entire date. Foreplay can even be many days of having met someone, time spent together and time spent apart. It can all be leading up to a sexual encounter where both parties are fully aware that they're leading up to it. So flirting, that's all foreplay. It doesn't need to be the actual physical intimacy. I think it should be very natural. My impulse is to move forward at a certain pace; that's my impulse. If the woman would want to go against that or prolong it that's her impulse and that's what creates the foreplay. Me holding myself back unnaturally to go through a certain number of steps, that seems like it could get contradictory. I think if the woman wants it prolonged, then she should prolong it and make it happen. It's really communicating.

BLASKO: I think it depends on the situation, but I'm into hanging out for a while before the deed gets done.

BRENT MUSCAT: With my girlfriends or any partners I've had, I sometimes like to do enough foreplay to make them come first so they get it out of the way and then no matter what you do… If you're Superman one night and you can last a long time, it's great, but if you're Quick Draw McGraw and you last two minutes, at least you've made them come and you've satisfied them and they're not disappointed. Of course, this is with someone you know; I don't know you'd want to do it with a stranger, but with someone you're dating. Going down on a girl enough to make them come, I think, is always a good thing. If you can make them come first, then if you're lucky, by the time you're having sex maybe they can have a second orgasm, two or three if you can get them into that state of arousal.

BRUCE KULICK: It all depends: if you're both really raring to go, you don't need a lot of it. I think it's hot when the second you check-in with your girl into your hotel room, you're tearing each other's clothes off. There's not a lot of foreplay but the foreplay is this whole concept of, 'We're going to tear up this hotel room!' I do think that on a typical romantic night though – you went to dinner, you had a little wine, you both look great, the conversation never went south where no one said anything stupid, no one's jealous, no one's pointing fingers or picking on each other and everything's just fun – obviously by the time it's ready to make the move on the couch or get into bed with them, you want to take your time and enjoy it and savour the moment and just kind of adore and worship your partner. That's foreplay to me.

CHIP Z'NUFF: Oh that's everything. If you're not a diner, you're not going to be a good lover. That starts the ball right away if you're going to get to the point where there's going to be sex. Dine, and that will start everything else up. Anything you're interested in doing after that will be much easier.

COURTNEY TAYLOR-TAYLOR: You just hope that whatever it is, it's exactly as much as keeps both of you there before one of you gets bored. That's how much. It depends on the situation and the people but for God's sake don't drag it out longer than the other person wants just because you're really having fun. Sometimes you can play that game for three hours ending in the most fucking wow orgasm of your life, or 34 minutes of whatever… it's just really all about where you're at and where they're at and just don't fuck it up. If you're fortunate enough to be in the situation where you are with another person that's interested in you sexually and you're interested in them, then chances are you're going to rush things anyway. But if you're in a serious relationship that's been going on for some time, then it becomes more like you're fortunate enough to be in a situation with a person that you're both sexually interested in at the same time, even though that's kind of your job. It's just very difficult later, particularly for men because we have so much caveman DNA driving us to impregnate a lot of different cavewomen. We've only been out of the cave for like 4,000 years and we've been around for like 100,000 or 300,000 years. So much of our programming is like women need to climb onto the most powerful ape in the cave and just dominate him so they can be protected in their pregnancy, then their child-bearing and the man (not even a man, but the man) is there. Then the man ape is just programmed to impregnate as many as we can in hopes that, you know, throw her against the wall and hope something sticks. So you've got an inherent problem in the relationship here. The motivations are different to begin with. It's almost always rare, except for the beginning, right at the front end of the relationship, to have two people that are both like, 'Fuck yeah' at the same time. Mostly, people I know are kind of single, alcoholic, good-looking, lonely and messed up. They get the most action because they're just lonely and they'll just do it. If they end up in bars they'll be with the best-looking guy or have the most going on – a little bit of notoriety with a local artist, filmmaker, musician, painter or something – they get the most action, but they're also super fucking lonely all the time. Coupled-up people, after the relationship has been on for a while, don't get much action, and single people that are alcoholics don't really get much action. Booze is a huge part of getting laid; sober people don't really score that much.

DANKO JONES: Forty minutes is good.

DOUG ROBB: It depends: sometimes you can just look at each other and go, 'It's fucking on, right now!' and no foreplay is needed, and sometimes lots of foreplay is good. I don't think foreplay is bad in any situation. I think most girls would agree with me and most guys would disagree with me. If it's going to help your girl get off in the end, then it's a little adjustment. It's not like going to the dentist or anything. So let's face it, the guys are going to get off either way; it doesn't matter, so why not put a little extra into it?

EVAN SEINFELD: That depends if it's with *your* partner or just with *a* partner, because the only woman I really like to give foreplay to is my wife, but she turns me on so much I'm popping and I just kind of ravage her. Foreplay is like my worst department ever. Foreplay has been a constant complaint; by the way, the *only* complaint I've had from partners in my life.

HANDSOME DICK MANITOBA: As much as possible.

JAMES KOTTAK: Whatever the chick wants. She's the boss.

JESSE HUGHES: The amount required, and that's a variable. Foreplay is sex too. The bizarre need to define it in two separate places is almost trippy. Sex is a thing that's just like music to me, man. We let the music tell us what it wants and we obey it and we try not to put too much or too little into it. The music is what you're making baby, you just let it tell you what to do; you know what I'm saying?

JIMMY ASHHURST: I've found that the more suspense that there is, the bigger the climax normally. So, the more the merrier – *if* you have the opportunity. Coming from a rock'n'roll standpoint, we seldom have that luxury; we're normally here for a good time, not a long time.

JOEL O'KEEFFE: Until you're out of the cold and warm and cosy inside.

LEMMY: Foreplay is the greatest part of sex; much better than the actual act. You can make foreplay last for a couple of days if you really care to.

NICKE BORG: Great foreplay is always good, so long as it doesn't become the most important thing in the whole sexual act. Foreplay is only like before play – we are talking about fucking right? Foreplay is not fucking. Foreplay is to get you excited. If you keep on fucking around during the foreplay for fucking ages, sooner or later she and you are obviously going to lose interest in having sex. So I think a little foreplay. But sometimes the foreplay is in your head and you can go right there, but you have to assess it from time to time depending on the situation you're in. Foreplay is always good but don't make it into, 'Hey, I can lick you for three hours.' You don't have to.

ROB PATTERSON: As much as you can take.

TOBY RAND: I love a lot of foreplay; probably 70% foreplay for me, because I think that with foreplay your eyes are kind of *there*. It actually depends on what kind of foreplay, but with using your hands and stuff like that where you're just caressing and shit… a lot of that – love it!

VAZQUEZ: I think it depends on how attracted you are to the person. I look at it this way: If I'm going to go down on a woman, or whatever, it's like I want her to have fun – I want her to feel good and usually if you get the pumps primed, so to speak, and you get her off one time before you really start fucking her, then you're going to walk away as the star, again!

What foreplay technique has them begging for more every time?

ACEY SLADE: Oral. I get the impression that a lot of guys aren't very good at oral, or don't even like it.

ADDE: A combination of talk and… it's really, really easy when you really, really are so hot for this woman. 'I'll do anything' and you do everything. That's probably the best way to really, really naturally feel it. 'I just want to satisfy this woman. I have a need for this', then anything goes.

BLASKO: Going down. You've got to use a combination of the fingers and the tongue whenever you're down there – that seems to work.

CHIP Z'NUFF: Dining while you're playing bass. Play bass. When you're dining, you just put a couple of fingers in and play bass guitar inside the pussy and you won't believe the things that happen there. I tell my friends about that, but you've got to practise before you can get good at that. I just run my fingers back and forth. I could be playing a Queen song, Jethro Tull, Grand Funk Railroad; it doesn't matter what song you play. Play bass the right way and they'll hail you forever.

DANKO JONES: I find making out and tit play. Does oral sex count as foreplay? That's not foreplay is it? I would not include that as foreplay and just say making out and tit play.

GINGER: Light conversation, based on her. Massage of the shoulders and back, not soft but not too hard. Once foreplay has begun then clitoral stimulation is a must, but don't allow her to cum until you have her in a state of sexual madness. She'll hate you for it at the time and remember you forever afterwards.

WHEN YOU'RE DINING, YOU JUST PUT A COUPLE OF FINGERS IN AND PLAY BASS GUITAR INSIDE THE PUSSY AND YOU WON'T BELIEVE THE THINGS THAT HAPPEN THERE.

HANDSOME DICK MANITOBA: Ladies first. As a man, you've always got to remember this: you are one second away from completely metamorphosing and losing your power – one second away. You've got to know that you can call on that second to always be there, it's always there waiting for you, and if you call on that second and you're just caring about yourself too much then you blow the whole thing. Also, there's a spiritual principle involved, which is you get by giving. Get into the thing of getting a lot of pleasure by giving, and know that your moment will come. And also know that if you don't control and own that moment, you're a bad lover.

JIMMY ASHHURST: If you're in the circumstance where you have access to toys and contraptions, any selection of those; the old vibrator is normally good. But in a pinch, the old fingers in the hands of a master. [Ed. Is that why they nicknamed you Two Fingers?] Very good, very good.

LEMMY: It depends on the girl and what she likes. You can do one thing to one girl and doing the same to another could get howls of outrage from the second, whereas the first one lapped it up. I think you're pretty safe with cunnilingus. That always goes down pretty well. Tying her to a boat and taking her out for a swim is always good too, because if you pull her out of the water she'll do anything.

ROB PATTERSON: That is a secret!

TOBY RAND: When the girl's lying on her stomach and you're above them and you're just kissing down their back and then kiss in between the ass and the back of their thighs. Then they want to move but you tell them to 'Shut up' and you hold them down.

VAZQUEZ: I don't really have any magic tricks in that sense but I think you've really got to ask the woman. There are women that just want you to touch their clit like so gently, and there are women that are like, 'Fucking bite it!' So, every woman is different. They're all different, which is part of why I guess we love them so much.

How can you extend foreplay when you're just busting to get it on?

ACEY SLADE: I let it rip and go again. Excuse yourself for a minute, take care of it, and get back on the horse… back on the bicycle.

ALLISON ROBERTSON: I think you can extend it if you figure out something that the other person likes. If neither party is bored I think you can extend it for quite a long time, but it all depends on the skills the two of you have. Some people just don't have any and it's like, 'Well this is boring. Let's just go to the next step.' I think if you have a skill of any kind, it doesn't matter what it is, that's how you can extend it by showing off a little bit.

BLASKO: I think you dive into getting it on and pull back. Then you kind of have a couple of times when you then go back into that.

CHIP Z'NUFF: You just have to. You just have to fight it and think about her because the more times she comes, the better you're going to receive that too. So take care of her for as long as you can until you're tired and then get ready for her to kick your ass because you just got it reciprocated. It always works. It's not like a small percentage, it always works.

DANKO JONES: There is a technique where we used the clock and we said, 'OK, we cannot start for half an hour. We have to just have foreplay for half an hour.' It would just make you do all kinds of crazy stuff and you'd have to think about what to do to kill the next ten minutes when everything's just going crazy. Usually we'd cut it short, but that would be the technique we'd use to extend it.

DOUG ROBB: I think when you're at that point of busting to get it on you should just get it on. You're done with the appetiser and it's time for the main course. Why would you continue to sit there and continue to eat the appetiser?

EVAN SEINFELD: I'm the wrong guy to ask. If you want to know what *not* to do, watch me.

JAMES KOTTAK: Think about Niagara Falls.

JESSE HUGHES: Be willing to go down. That will extend foreplay any old day of the week.

JIMMY ASHHURST: Patience is a virtue, man. If you can keep in mind that the payout's going to be better for the both of you and the chance for a second date will be increased a lot. I think impatience is the mark of an immature soul; the longer you can hang out the better.

LEMMY: Well that's a matter of self control. I like a bit of self control. The longer you keep that going the less time you have actually fucking; you realise that?

ROB PATTERSON: Take breaks; don't stay on one part for too long. Make it last.

TOBY RAND: You hold them down. You seriously hold them down. I think the best thing about sex is the anticipation of not knowing when it's all going to happen. That's why foreplay's great.

Have you found a correlation between foreplay time and orgasm quality?

ACEY SLADE: Oh, for sure! Definitely the longer the foreplay, the more intense the orgasm. There's a girl that I tied up one time and made her watch porn movies for two hours while I had foreplay with her.

ADDE: Yeah, absolutely! It's all in the foreplay.

ALLISON ROBERTSON: No, I actually haven't. I don't think there is a correlation between that, at least not for me. I think that it completely depends on all kinds of things, like how long it's been since the last time whoever had sex, how everything fits together in the puzzle pieces, how hot it is outside or how cold. I think all that stuff changes everything and I don't think it matters how much foreplay.

ANDREW W.K.: For sure and that's really the thing to keep in mind I guess, but not necessarily the amount of time before the actual intercourse or when the actual sexual interaction starts. I think just being sexual for a long time will increase the quality of the orgasm; holding back basically. It doesn't need to be leading up for hours of kissing, you can begin your sex but the longer you wait, the better the orgasm will be – always; it's never not gone that way. But, sometimes you can wait too long and then lose it. That's really a bummer, because you've held out, you've held out, you've held out, then it's almost like your body says, 'OK, fine. If you don't want to come then that's it.' There's only so much stamina that one person could have and you at least hope you can get the reward of the orgasm at the end, but many people say it's not always about the orgasm. If you can keep it feeling good… there are sexual techniques to make the entire time you're having sex feel like the orgasm basically. It's not like literally you're having an orgasm that whole time, but you're in such control that it's not about leading up to that uncontrollable part.

BLASKO: I've never paid much attention to that – interesting theory though.

BRENT MUSCAT: Each girl is different: some girls can orgasm in a minute or two whereas some girls will take like 20 minutes. And there are some girls I've experienced that – I don't know how, maybe they won't let themselves go – but they can't come and they will tell you that they've never come before with anybody, which is a little bizarre, but I think it's mental. I think there's that old saying that most of sex is really in between your ears; it's in your mind. It's a rare occasion that you find someone that just can't let go enough to orgasm.

BRUCE KULICK: I do think that some foreplay will certainly go a long way, rather than none. I do know that if you're both raring to go, you don't need the foreplay and there could be orgasms galore. So it's all relative to how hot the moment is.

COURTNEY TAYLOR-TAYLOR: It's quality and quality I think. Sometimes it's just getting off and a question of intensity. Time is irrelevant.

DANKO JONES: Oh yeah! Yeah, definitely more foreplay and at the end a greater orgasm. The more intense the orgasm for sure; that's definitely a correlation there.

DOUG ROBB: Yeah, I think the longer the anticipation and the longer the build-up, the more rewarding it'll probably be.

EVAN SEINFELD: Absolutely, I think the longer it takes for me to come, the better the orgasm is. It's also fighting the animal instincts to fuck and come, so it's difficult. I have some really great orgasms when I do porn scenes because I'm fucking for an hour and a half or two hours without coming. But still, the most intense orgasm I ever have is when my wife just lays me back and knows exactly how to handle me.

HANDSOME DICK MANITOBA: I think there's a direct correlation, yes. I don't want to generalise, but generally you have two different kinds of animals: the female animal and male animal. They're both coming at sex from different angles. It seems like it's more of a physical animal experience with the males and it's more of a total experience with the females. So the more you acknowledge that totality and put time and effort in and build up, then it seems that women get to the point where they're male-like, in terms of them becoming like animals also.

JAMES KOTTAK: None.

JESSE HUGHES: Quality of the orgasm is a direct result of the amount of input and enthusiasm put into it by the male. Almost generally, because from the outset a woman feels you don't care about her orgasm, the second you put any enthusiastic attempts directly and specifically to her orgasm, it will make her go bang in a bigger way by virtue of the fact that she feels like you're doing something extra. It's the easiest thing to do and it's the last thing he ever thinks of doing because it's just like a power struggle, but it's so lame. Sorry, I believe in that.

QUALITY OF THE ORGASM IS A DIRECT RESULT OF THE AMOUNT OF INPUT AND ENTHUSIASM PUT INTO IT BY THE MALE.

LEMMY: No, I don't think so. Sometimes you feel like thrusting and you're gone before you get inside her. Other times you're banging away and she says, 'Fucking hell, stop! I'm sore.' There's no way of telling.

ROB PATTERSON: Absolutely. The longer you hold out, the harder and better it is!

TOBY RAND: Definitely! The more foreplay the better the orgasm – hands down. The more you hold off, the better – even for the girl as well.

VAZQUEZ: I think it just comes down to what they want; I always ask them what they want. I think most women really dig that because they're like, 'Oh OK, cool – he gets it.' If you give them exactly what they want, they love it. I've been with girls who are like, 'I've never been able to get off with a guy fucking me' and I'm like, 'Hey, well then they just didn't listen to you.' It's great to be that guy because man, you own them.

Is there a good way to get aroused if you're not really in the mood?

ACEY SLADE: There's always the back catalogue of events that you have in your head. I usually resort to them.

ADDE: Talk dirty to me, like Poison said. Talk dirty to me, yeah. And talk really, really dirty.

ALLISON ROBERTSON: I think that if you have a good imagination you can get excited about anything. If you're with somebody who you don't really like that much or whatever, or just distracted, I think if you have a good imagination you can focus on a fantasy or something like that, maybe from an older time in your life when sex was better or whatever. I think it's sad if you have to dig into the archives, or as Larry David would say you have to go to the bench – that's like the line-up of people who he has fantasies about. I think it's kind of sad if you're with someone longer than once or twice and you have to keep doing that, thinking about other things, but I think that's a way to help if you're having trouble.

BLASKO: I don't know that there is – if you aren't into it, you aren't into it.

BRENT MUSCAT: For me, I think if the girl goes down on you and gives you a blowjob that usually works. If you're not really in the mood, I think you can still get there. Maybe there's something bothering you, maybe you need a hot bath, maybe a glass of wine or something, or if you've got a headache take an aspirin. I've never really had the problem of not being able to get in the mood.

BRUCE KULICK: Oh, I always think that if a girl grabs my dick or goes down on me that will get me aroused. Generally I'm never not in the mood, but if there's an occasion where I wasn't for whatever reason, like I might have been very wound up or just stressed about business or whatever, I can get out of that fairly quickly. The only time I've ever had the issue of like, 'I'm just not into it' is clearly when I've just been so overly exhausted. Now I know to avoid that.

Why would I want to have sex? Just to say I did it? Sometimes I surprise myself by acting like a 20-year-old. I feel happy for me and proud of my partner that she turns me on like that.

CHIP Z'NUFF: Yeah, but a lot of women don't like to hear about it. That would be thinking about past experiences and what quality times you've had with exes that may have been really great. You might have had great chemistry with them and it always worked out really well, and if you think back to that it'll help you but don't ever tell them that; that's for sure. I think your best bet is to just bite the bullet and still take care of them first. It solves everything; it really does. If you're just a selfish guy that just wants to bone all the time, that's not going to work for you. But if you're not in the mood but she is, dine, play some bass, and that'll help her because once she gets off a few times she doesn't care if you nail her or not after that.

DANKO JONES: Porn.

JAMES KOTTAK: Go down!

JIMMY ASHHURST: Masturbation usually works. Also try YouPorn.com – it's fucking free and it's amazing.

LEMMY: I feel a cattle prod in the asshole will usually do it.

NICKE BORG: You probably have some kind of mental disease or something if you have a beautiful girl asking – basically begging – you to fuck her. I'm not into sports and shit, but I have this friend and, with the hockey finals now, she broke up with him. So I would never say, 'There are hockey finals on now, so can we make out in two hours?' Fuck that; fuck the hockey finals dude, but that's me.

ROB PATTERSON: Put on some kinky shit on the TV. Ha.

TOBY RAND: Headjob. One word.

VAZQUEZ: If a woman is with me and she's naked, I'm happy, man – I'm aroused.

GROUPIES

"THE WILDEST GROUPIES:
ENGLAND. THE HOTTEST
GROUPIES: AUSTRALIA"

What's the best and worst thing about groupies?

ACEY SLADE: Groupies. The best thing and the worst thing about groupies is groupies.

ADDE: The best thing is that they are around, all over the world – the whole world. It's a really, really good thing for a musician to have. They're a musician's best friend. The worst thing is the phone calls.

ALLISON ROBERTSON: The good thing about groupies is that they're there and they support you in your actual job. I think the difference between a male groupie and a female groupie is this: if I were a guy, I would probably continue to say the other good thing about groupies is that they're willing to do whatever, they're hot, they're well-groomed or usually they try to be looking their best, they're really submissive and they're kind of like pets. But because we're girls, we get a lot of guys who are more like a male groupie, but the thing is they aren't always well-groomed and they're not always hot. If there were a bunch of guys lined up outside our dressing room who were wearing hot business suits, had really great bodies, or were wearing just a banana hammock and tanned and oiled, that would be the equivalent of what Mötley Crüe get outside their room, or at least back in the Eighties. I've never seen that. Once in a while you'll see a hot guy in the audience or something and then they always disappear. The bad thing about male groupies is that a lot of them are aggressive, they don't smell good, and they have no tact or no game. It's the complete opposite of a girl who's flirty and smells nice and has her boobs pushed up. I can see why a guy in a band would think that would be great. I can totally see why that would be appealing, but it's very different for females to find that kind of something on the road I think.

ANDREW W.K.: The best thing is getting attention. Being desired is a great feeling. That's very primal: wanting affection, wanting to be cared for, wanting someone to love you, to think that you're important. That's a great feeling and that's an opportunity that the groupie world presents for both sides: to be desired as the fan and to be desired as the object of adoration. But the groupies, I think they really want that fair trade where they want to feel important at that time, whether it's importance through being desired by the band member, the importance of being let into the band member's world, the exclusivity, getting to see the inside, to just the gall, the nerve, the courage it takes to try to go backstage or on the bus or to be intimate. So it's a real trade. I guess one way it could be looked at is the band wants to have sex and they're exchanging access into this cool world that the groupie's interested in.

BLASKO: The best thing about them is that they exist. The worst thing about them is that they exist.

BRENT MUSCAT: The best thing is they're a lot of fun – a ton of fun! They're usually into partying and there's nothing wrong with it. A lot of people look down on groupies. I really tip my hat to them and respect them. If a girl wants to go out and have fun, then why not? Because guys do it. A guy in a band can go from every town and screw a different girl each night and he doesn't really get labelled as a slut. So in some ways I don't think it's fair to even say groupies as a derogatory term like, 'Oh, she's just a groupie.' I'm like, 'Man, that's a good thing. Thank God for groupies! Imagine how boring and how lonely it would be if you had to tour if you had no female companionship for months?' So, I think groupies are great. The best thing is that they're there and they're willing to party and stuff. The worst thing might be when sometimes they like to brag and it can get you in trouble, especially nowadays with the internet. When I first started touring, if you were on tour in Japan, or you were in another country, you could have the time of your life and your girlfriend back home would never know anything. But now with the internet, I guess the worst thing about groupies is they love to brag about their conquests.

BRUCE KULICK: Obviously the ones that are very catty and sloppy and can really be outright rude to the girls around them, that's the worst of the groupies. I can even respect, 'Oh Def Leppard's in town this week so I slept with this guy or that guy. Kiss is in town next week; I'm going to sleep with this guy or that guy.' I get that. That's OK. If you can be like in the movie *Almost Famous* – a Band-Aid – meaning you're truly making that musician feel welcome and that what he does makes a difference with all that touring and everything. 'I'm here to just thank you and adore you and maybe fuck you', then I think that's the best part of the groupie scene. Now unfortunately, you do get a lot of broken people doing that, who need to do that. No one's good enough in their home town so they seek out band members or they're so hot that they can't help it. They figure, 'Oh I can get him, so I may as well.' There have been many girls, like Pamela Des Barres who wrote the book (I don't know her in any intimate way) who clearly knew how to play that better role and not that obnoxious, crazy role that some groupies do. Some of them are really screwed up and unfortunately either the drugs or that need for attention is not a healthy thing.

CHIP Z'NUFF: Every time I meet girls they always say, 'I'm not a groupie', but I just shrug that off because I know that's not true. The best thing about groupies is they love the band. They're good for our egos. It's essential and they've been around for years and years and years before us. It's something that started up in the Twenties and Thirties with the vaudeville bands and big band stuff; there were groupies back then. The worst thing about them is they carry certain things that we don't want and they talk too much. They're not very discreet and that's questionable right there.

COURTNEY TAYLOR-TAYLOR: The best thing about groupies is that they exist and the worst thing is that it's a cliché.

DANKO JONES: It's a great ego boost to know there are girls/women who are interested in you just by the music and they've seen your photo or whatever. That's a great ego boost. How many jobs get that? It's a great perk that's nice for the ego. There's always a dark side to it because sometimes people who hang out all the way to the very end of the night, who just want to be with someone they don't know but think they do, sometimes (not all the time; sometimes people are pretty genuine) those people have a screw loose or something; I don't know. They bring a lot of drama, let's put it that way. They tend to bring a lot of drama and drama is something I've tried to get out of my life. When I sense it now, I immediately avoid it. So it's good and bad and I've just noticed from the sidelines too, when I took myself out of that whole thing and I just said, 'I can't really do this and continue on', you just watch other guys do it and see the whole drama unfold and it's pretty much by the book, by the numbers – the drama unfolding, the non-stop phone calls. I just think you don't need that. It can be a great thing; I wish that every groupie could look like Kylie Minogue or Heather Graham, but it's just not like that all the time.

DOUG ROBB: The best thing about groupies is watching the Walk of Shame. That's when you're sitting in the front of the bus and one of your band members is in the back of the bus and it's time to go, and this random chick comes out of the back lounge and reassembles her dishevelled self to try and make it look like nothing was going on. We'll all be sitting in the front and they'll walk by and they'll act as hard as they can to make it look like nothing happened and they're not that type of girl or whatever. We're all smiling and being polite. The bus door will close and we'll all start laughing and we'll look down the hall and here comes whoever from the back, like, 'Smell my finger'. So that's a source of a lot of laughter. The worst thing about groupies is – I see them more often than not – groupies are probably the least attractive women; they're pretty horrible.

EVAN SEINFELD: One of the best things about groupies is that they provide a service. They're there to make a band's life on the road easier and it's part of the fruits of our labour. I've been a rock musician for 20-plus years and I've been an actor for 10. And I'll say this: when you're working on a feature film or a TV series, you form a great team, but when you're done there usually aren't girls waiting there to blow you. But I've got to say the best thing about it is the nameless, thankless blowjob where they feel they owe it to you because they are groupies and you deserve it; you performed a concert. It's part of your rite of passage as a rock star is that you put on a great show, somebody should suck your dick! That's why you became a rock star in the first place – it wasn't for the money.

The worst thing about it is when they want to talk to you and tell you all the other guys they're friends with. There are three things when you know a girl's a groupie – I'm making this up right now: 1) When they ask you if you know blank from so-and-so band. He might be in the band or he might just be a roadie. 'Do you know so-and-so from this band? He's a really good friend of mine' and you're a groupie and I'm turned off. 2) Right as she puts your dick in her mouth, she looks up at you and says, 'I've never done anything like this before.' This is 99% across the board from real groupies. They feel obligated to pretend that they're not a slut, which kind of blows my mind because I kind of want you to be a slut. I want you to say, 'I suck every cock that comes through town because I love rock stars and I'm here to give you the best blowjob you've ever had.' It'd be better than, 'I've not done this before.' 3) The third thing can be when they are what we call a good sport. Are they going to blow everybody else in the bus, band, crew and the bus driver? Because you know, bus drivers need love too!

HANDSOME DICK MANITOBA: It's a tough one. We weren't a band that just like, you know… some bigger bands had groupies outside and stuff… I'm a strange guy that way: I'd meet girls on the road and I'd like them enough to be comfortable with them and fool around with them, but I *liked* them. I had very, very few experiences where it was like, 'Give me some head.' I had a couple of those and I didn't find any problems or anything negative about it. Then there were a few where people liked my band and I'd hang out with them and have sex with them, go see a movie with them, have dinner with them and have sex with them again and I kind of like that – I kind of like that more than just, 'Let's get some bitches to suck our dicks!' That wasn't big in my life. Only occasional moments where I'm like, 'God damn, I'm horny! Suck my dick!' It wasn't a day-to-day routine, let's put it that way.

I WISH THAT EVERY GROUPIE COULD LOOK LIKE KYLIE MINOGUE OR HEATHER GRAHAM, BUT IT'S JUST NOT LIKE THAT ALL THE TIME.

JAMES KOTTAK: The best thing is getting the free massages. The worst thing is when they smell.

JESSE HUGHES: That they come back is the worst thing and the best thing is that it's usually hot sex. But I don't really believe in the concept of the groupie. To me, I like to go to rock shows with rock'n'rollers and I get down with my kind. That's the way I look at it and it definitely improves the game.

JIMMY ASHHURST: The worst thing is when they try and convince you that they're not groupies. The best thing is when they try and convince you that they're not groupies.

JOEL O'KEEFFE: The best thing is they generally always 'put out' in one way or another. The worst thing is when their boyfriend or Dad shows up – then it's time for The Great Escape!

LEMMY: Well the best thing is that they're up for anything and the worst thing is that they follow you after going down to breakfast in the hotel. You have to hope the crew left already, or you've never heard the last of it.

NICKE BORG: Groupies is an interesting word in general because it has such a fucking negative ring to it, and I don't think of them as a negative thing. It's the same kind of negative thing as if you say this is a rock ballad – no, it's a slow song. So I see groupies as fans who happen to be female (and I would hope that they are singles) and they see this person that they are so fucking attracted to because of the way he plays music and also the way he looks. Sometimes you can be sexy just by playing a good song, or you can look good and play a shit song, whatever. They're just like, 'I want to fuck him' and that's fine. I think that real fans that are just in it for the music really look down on these girls who love the music but also want to have that guy's cock in their whatever. And I'm like, 'What the fuck? It's a free world. Do whatever, man!' I think in sports there are even more groupies. But it just happens to be rock'n'roll music, girls wearing a short skirt and flash their tits at a show, and then they fuck the band in the dressing room – that's an old way of looking at it you know. So I would say for me that groupies are my fans. They're great; I love them!

ROB PATTERSON: Believe it or not, I've never had sex with a groupie!

TOBY RAND: The best thing is that you can have sex on tap… blowjobs. The worst thing is that they think they have an automatic ticket to be everywhere you go after that and you have to get rid of them. Enter security guards.

VAZQUEZ: This is what it comes down to: I've never really had a groupie that became a problem. The reason is because of The Two D's: Diplomacy and Discretion. I explain to them what my situation is and what they can expect, so that way I'm being completely upfront with them and they don't become psychos. I know dudes in bands who've had to change their fucking phone number every couple of months and it's like, 'Dude!' They do this shit when they're fucking hammered and they're fucking these girls and they're like, 'I love you' and saying all kinds of dumb shit and that's what fucks you. I'm always sober, I'm always honest and I've never had a problem. Diplomacy and discretion, man – that's what it's all about.

Should groupies expect sex if invited back to a band's hotel?

ACEY SLADE: Yeah, especially if she paid for the room.

ADDE: Yeah they should, they should.

ALLISON ROBERTSON: I think so! I'm really careful with someone I don't know or whatever. I'm doing this interview but I think everybody calls me prude. I've also been married and had a lot of long-term relationships so I've barely dabbled with anything on the road. But I have to say that yes, I think if you're invited back to a hotel room you should hope for it, unless you do something drastically wrong. That definitely happens with our band. I think if you're not invited back to the hotel that's a bad sign, but once you're invited then you're in – usually.

ANDREW W.K.: No, they shouldn't, they shouldn't, thank God! When I first started touring, I got freaked out a lot of times by the groupie scene and just how intense it was. It really is like in the movies. I was really shocked to see how much that existed and that there really are all these girls going around who are just ready to go. But I also saw a lot of times with people in my band and crew on big tours, that guys just want female companionship. They want to be around women for a change from being around a huge crew of often sweaty, close-quartered dudes. It's very nice to have female energy around. That was a really beautiful part about it because I think that a lot of the groupies also go in that way as well. You can flirt and you can be affectionate and maybe sometimes it'll be sexually on, but a lot of times it was just hanging out and wanting to be social with women. I thought that was a really cool part of it. I never really did much of it either way; I was just freaked out by the whole thing. I was just too shy to talk to people I didn't really know, especially women, and nowadays it's just a different vibe.

BLASKO: I would think so… not always, but if that's the mutual intention, then by all means.

BRENT MUSCAT: I don't think they should expect it, but maybe they should plan for it in case – bring some condoms. If that's what they're there for, at least be ready for it. Maybe being on the pill and having condoms would not be a bad thing, but I don't think they should expect it. I was in England one time and one of the girls came back and was kind of disappointed because nobody would have sex with her. It was like she was almost so desperate it was unattractive. She got kind of mad. She was like, 'What kind of band are you? What kind of rock guys are you?' There are also days when the guys are tired out, or not in the mood, or could be sick.

CHIP Z'NUFF: Some do, it depends. There's a difference between being a groupie and a Band-Aid of course. Band-Aids just love the music. Groupies want a little bit more to remember and you'll know the difference when you meet them. If it's a groupie, she'll immediately come out into the room and she'll be initiating it, whereas a Band-Aid will just hang out, just wants to listen to you talk, learn about you and spend quality time with you while you're in town, because they know you're going to be leaving in a few hours.

COURTNEY TAYLOR-TAYLOR: No, that's a personal thing. Guys in bands are pretty clear if they want one. If they're amateurs or whatever they'll make the mistake of getting a couple or many interested and end up with nothing. Expect sex? No, but if it's a group thing that's obviously why they or someone in their clique has been invited back to the hotel. I don't think that all of them end up getting some action, unless you can talk yourself into a group rate.

DANKO JONES: I think they kind of should but I don't think the band should expect sex. It gets to be a very weird, grey, touchy situation when the band is expecting it but they don't necessarily have a confirmation that the parties invited are expecting it as well. Then it gets to be really weird. That's another element of that whole thing that I've taken myself out of. It's very dangerous for both parties involved when there could be a misunderstanding. It's such a time-honoured tradition in pop culture that the band sometimes goes, 'Well don't you know? You should know! This is part of the tradition' and maybe it's just some real genuine person who really just wants to be around the band that he or she really likes. So it gets really touchy and I've seen it when a band – not necessarily our band – but a band has invited people on their bus or in their hotel room and you just look at them and go, 'Do they really know? Do both parties know what the other is thinking?' You just don't know. I think everything should be on the table. I think it should really be on the table when you invite someone up to your hotel room or when you invite someone onto the bus. Everything should be up front. It might be considered crass or vulgar, but in that situation I think it's the only way. Like a simple, 'Do you want to go upstairs and fuck?' might sound crass to everybody but I think you have to do that.

DOUG ROBB: Yeah, I think so because I think the hotel is like their house and they sure aren't inviting you back to play cards.

EVAN SEINFELD: Why else would you go to a guy's hotel in the middle of the night? I always hated that kind of game that a lot of girls play, this fake anti-presumptuous thing where it's like, 'Oh, why would you think that we were going to have sex?' 'I don't know. Every other girl who came to my hotel room in the last 20 years in the middle of the night had sex with me, why would I think you were any different?' A lot of girls think they're different and they want to think they're like girlfriend material – ladies, be glad you're enjoying having sex with us tonight.

HANDSOME DICK MANITOBA: Yeah. I think there are groupies in every aspect of life. Up by the police station near my house there's women hanging around. There are women that hang around all kinds of uniforms. Rock'n'roll is just another uniform.

JAMES KOTTAK: Not with me, but anybody else. Go for it. I encourage it.

JESSE HUGHES: Yeah! It ain't no fucking Bible study. When you go to church, you pretty much know what to expect. You *can* judge a book by its cover. You buy fucking *Hustler* you know what you're getting. You buy *Good Housekeeping* you know what that is. That ain't no fucking mystery. When you come home with a rock'n'roller, you'd better fucking believe they're going to expect you're getting down.

JIMMY ASHHURST: They should, absolutely.

JOEL O'KEEFFE: Yes, otherwise why would the band invite them back, especially if their drugs and booze are limited? They're not going to take freeloaders unless they're going to free their loads!

LEMMY: Well I imagine so, yeah. Mind you: Mike Tyson; that should be a sobering reminder to us all. I never insisted it on a chick that didn't want it. I never did that. I always tried to be within the decencies of a decent person.

NICKE BORG: I once invited a girl back to my room because she didn't know who The Cult was. So obviously I had to fucking go to the bus, pull up my iTunes and play 'Electric' by The Cult so she would understand that they are one of the greatest bands in the world. And that's it – nothing else – I swear to fucking God! So it depends on person to person; sometimes sitting down and having a nice conversation with someone you never met before, but you just realised that you have a lot in common with that person, is sometimes so much better than sex.

ROB PATTERSON: From what I hear from old bandmates, yes.

TOBY RAND: Yes. But sometimes they come in groups, so if you want the one you want, she might bring some friends – so for them, no.

VAZQUEZ: I would definitely say no, because some dudes, they just don't do it. Some dudes just want a blowjob, some dudes just want to talk, man.

How can a groupie best attract the attention of a rock star?

ACEY SLADE: For the most part, you've got to be an attractive girl. You have to start off there. You can't look too desperate. You still have to have that confidence.

ADDE: For me, it's to not be a rock chick. Be like a disguised groupie, like 'I'm a librarian' and look like a librarian. That's the thing for me, but I think 90% of all the rock stars go for, 'Oh, she's hot for me, I'll fuck her!', whereas I'm like, 'I want the one at the back.'

ALLISON ROBERTSON: I think with groupies you want to look the best; not that it's all about looks, but if you're in a crowd obviously you're going to stand out if you look good. But I also think by not looking desperate. Especially with females, no women really want to go for a guy that seems desperate; it's not sexy. It's especially cool when someone's a little more confident and seems like fun, because at the end of the day, obviously you're not looking to get married if you're on the road and you meet somebody. You're looking for someone who's fun, easy-going and seems like they're a good kisser. As far as all my female friends go, that would be what would make a guy groupie stand out.

BRENT MUSCAT: Wearing something sexy probably, being friendly, being attractive and acting cool. Someone who's not acting too desperate.

DANKO JONES: I say look really fucking hot! It always works.

GINGER: Don't attract the attention of anyone but the person you plan on getting close to. You can be friendly with the rest of the band and crew after you've bagged your star and been invited back.

JAMES KOTTAK: Blonde, big boobs.

JESSE HUGHES: Be hot! It's the best way to attract the attention. It's that clichéd and it's absolutely that frivolous.

JIMMY ASHHURST: Coming with the right number of people is important. I've found that pairs, as in duos, is not quite as good because in order for the doer to be split up, the other one has to find something else to do. You have to have a bandmate or someone else to take one aside – that whole wingman situation. Now, more than three is a drag too because they're usually party girls and it's very difficult to separate one from the pack. So I've found that trios are the perfect number because you can drag one and the other two can spend the rest of the night talking shit about what a slut that one is.

JOEL O'KEEFFE: With a coy smile and a wink, or if that doesn't work, spike his drink! I didn't mind the last time my drink was spiked, as I was having a shit night but then all of a sudden I was having the best night of my life and spent the entire night at the hospital playing in a children's castle.

LEMMY: Taking her top off in the audience will easily do it if she's got nice tits.

NICKE BORG: Not being in the first row flashing her tits, banging her head against the barricade and having a bleeding wound on her forehead and at the same time screaming, 'I want to suck your cock!' That could be very interesting to look at in a way, but there's something wrong with that person… and she probably knows that too. Ha! Dude, just be cool. Don't go on about rare 7" vinyl singles; don't flash your tits out. Just be like, 'Hey, I love your fucking shit. You're cool. Do you want to have a drink? I'm in the bar you know, back there. When you're done after your show, if you want to come, I'll buy you a drink.' Then it's just like a normal pickup line, like you do in general.

ROB PATTERSON: Introduce themselves.

TOBY RAND: I've found that I love the ones that are reserved, yet confident. They don't overstep the mark. They'll come up and say something cool and leave it up to me. I don't want to be forced into something or have pressure put on. I think a bit of control for us is good.

VAZQUEZ: Direct eye contact, definitely, and don't be fucking shy. Fuck that – I hate shy.

How can a wannabe groupie get backstage?

ACEY SLADE: MySpace has made it so much easier, so groupies can bypass the whole old roadies thing of if you hook up with a roadie you can get backstage. Well if I knew that she was with a roadie, then I definitely wouldn't be with that girl – if I knew that I was getting sloppy seconds. But one thing that is kind of funny about MySpace now is everybody's accessible, so it's not too hard to meet a band guy online, talk them up, chat them up, get on the guest list and he knows you're there.

BLASKO: Generally, it's like working your way through the crew, working your way through a guitar tech, bass tech – the immediate guy. Not the rigger, not the dude who's the assistant to the front of house guy. It's got to be like the onstage guys.

DOUG ROBB: I would say just look as attractive as possible and be cool. Just flirt with guys. It's the same way those groupies get into clubs, you know. They go up to the bouncer and act a little aloof… whatever, I don't know. Girls know what they're doing.

JOEL O'KEEFFE: Pick-pocket a pussy pass or be daring enough to do whatever it takes. One piece of valuable information: the more hardcore groupies seem to have learned that there is always a load-in/band entrance to every venue and it's always unlocked so the roadies can go out and smoke with ease. Give a roadie a 'smoke' and he just might give you everything you came for.

NOT TOO MANY OF THEM WANT TO BE BACKSTAGE AT A MOTÖRHEAD SHOW. WE'RE TOO OLD AND FUCKING UGLY NOW.

LEMMY: Not too many of them want to be backstage at a Motörhead show. We're too old and fucking ugly now. You can get backstage if you want to get backstage; chicks aren't without resources. You don't need to read your book to get backstage.

ROB PATTERSON: Well, like I said, I can only go from stories I've heard. Talk a roadie into giving them a pass. If you're hot, it won't be that hard.

TOBY RAND: From what I've seen, you go through the road crew and then most of the groupies will get picked on and laughed at by the band. They make it all the way through to the band and the band goes, 'Didn't you just sleep with the stage guy?' and they go, 'Why the fuck would you sleep with that guy?'

VAZQUEZ: They usually just wait around, they do The Wait. You're like loading out and you see them kind of just hanging around, standing there.

What city in the world has the wildest groupies?

ACEY SLADE: Wildest? I don't know about cities, but definitely Germany and England. They're kind of up for anything; anything goes with groupies in England or Germany.

ADDE: Probably in Italy because we play there so much. They really, really know what they want. They're really like, 'Arrgghhh'… aggressive.

ALLISON ROBERTSON: I think the South in the US. There are a lot of rowdy, confident, cute guys there. I think in general the people there are good, girls too; everybody's just really festive. I also think whenever we've been to Australia, there are a lot of cute guys and they're nice and they're friendly and it's not like in LA, where there's a lot of hot guys who are really douche bags. In Australia and in New Zealand – we did the Big Day Out festival – I remember we did a show and there were all these people from New Zealand at the signing and everybody was hunky. They all would have been invited back to the hotel room. A good warm vibe, that's what you want. You don't want a bunch of weirdos that seem like they're on drugs or tripping out. So I think generally, it's best when you're in a spot where it's warmer weather, good-looking people, and everybody likes rock'n'roll, so maybe Brazil too; there are hot guys in Brazil.

ANDREW W.K.: The vibe in Latin America was very intense. The girls there were really talking about wanting to get married and they would do anything. There was a level of… I won't say desperate because it didn't come off as desperate, it just came off as way, way, way more intense. Like, I thought the fans in Japan were intense but it wasn't until Mexico that I saw this other level of intensity. It's just a very passionate culture and the devotional quality of some of the girls there and the way they sort of offered themselves, there was no cat and mouse game going on, it was just here I am.

BRENT MUSCAT: Salt Lake City, Utah. The Mormon girls – I don't know what it is but they're pretty wild. They're very good-looking, tall, big and just blonde. Not that I'm totally into blondes, but it's kind of like a nice change of pace when you go in their city and you're like, 'Woah!' These blonde Amazon women with their bodies, they look great; very healthy looking.

CHIP Z'NUFF: New York: it's open 24 hours, everything goes and it's just one of those cities unlike any other. However, LA is right up there with New York. Like I said, they have those big, huge parties with the ecstasy and the Viagra and the cocaine – strawberry cocaine by the way; that's the big thing now. I prefer New York myself. I just like the way they carry themselves and I just love the city. It never stops. LA does stop. Things close up out there. New York is 24 hours. It's probably my favourite city in the whole world for everything. We're playing there tonight. It's a Mecca. The greatest bands go there, they play the biggest shows. It's wonderful being at Madison Square Gardens. You've got the Radio City Music Hall, Irving Plaza, really good venues to play out there. You meet quality people and there's just a plethora of trim.

COURTNEY TAYLOR-TAYLOR: Athens, Greece maybe. Probably next is going to be like Adelaide, Australia. Yeah Adelaide is still kind of a Wild West town. Perth, Australia is really cool; I wouldn't say those groupies are really wild. The chicks that hang out with bands in Perth are kind of smart and cool and fun actually. Oslo, Norway too.

DANKO JONES: There's been some crazy nights and then you go back and it's not as crazy. Countries I could probably tell you: England, Germany.

DOUG ROBB: I think college towns in the States. I wouldn't consider them groupies, but they're just young and most of the time really drunk and kind of oblivious. They just go crazy. They're kind of busy trying to prove to the next girl that they're crazy and rock'n'roll. It's funny to kind of watch them compete over groupiness.

EVAN SEINFELD: It's got to be a toss-up between Detroit, Cleveland and Buenos Aires, Argentina.

HANDSOME DICK MANITOBA: My guess would be LA.

JAMES KOTTAK: I would definitely have to say Los Angeles.

JESSE HUGHES: The wildest groupies: England. The hottest groupies: Australia.

JIMMY ASHHURST: Any city in Canada, oddly enough. Maybe it's something to do with the cold and that most of the guys are just interested in hockey and beer.

LEMMY: Best time I ever had I think was Argentina. And Japan. The first time in Japan was fantastic. The second time we went back not much happened. Third time it was great again, so it depends.

NICKE BORG: Florida, in general. America in general of course, but there's kind of something weird about Japan. They can be like, 'I think rock stars expect all women to be sluts so we dress like sluts and if you want to fuck us, you can fuck us, and we like your music very much' you know? It's like, 'What the fuck are you talking about?' Weird. I think the whole groupie thing was like England and America; it was invented there in a way.

ROB PATTERSON: Hmm… I think Russia, maybe?

TOBY RAND: I think Vancouver is awesome. Florida, as a state. Buffalo. I don't know… there's just so many. I think that groupies are wild everywhere.

VAZQUEZ: I'd have to say a cross between LA and Japan. It's apples and oranges, but for the United States I think the girls in LA are fucking great.

HYGIENE & GROOMING

"I THINK A WOMAN SHOULD HAVE NO HAIR ON HER BODY FROM HER EYEBROWS DOWN"

How much pubic hair should be left on ladies for maximum turn-on?

ACEY SLADE: I think a woman should have no hair on her body from her eyebrows down. Eyebrows are optional (tattooed eyebrows are gross).

ADDE: I say leave it all on. Bring back the Seventies – the Seventies bush baby!

ALLISON ROBERTSON: Oh I think women should have a little something down there. I've always thought that. I think almost all my hot girlfriends and everybody I know, everybody agrees, as far as in the rock'n'roll world. I've always thought that, but everybody has their own taste. I think girls should do what they want to do. I know a lot of girls who are like, 'Oh my boyfriend likes it completely bare,' and I'm like, 'When did that happen?' It's just a trend. I like the old *Playboy* magazines where there's a little more going on down there. I think as long as you're well-groomed and it's not frightening, it's nice to be a little natural. I think everything on women and men should be as natural as possible.

ANDREW W.K.: It depends on how she maintains it, but I'm fine with none, or like zero to five.

BLASKO: Not a whole lot, pretty minimal. The little patch can differ occasionally or evolve to a little landing strip. They can get creative every now and then you know, but that's about the extent of it.

BRENT MUSCAT: I think they should be trimmed, at least. I think the Seventies bush is bad and a bunch of hair down the legs is kind of gross. I think a nice waxing would be good and just trimmed I think is sexy. I think a little strip of hair always looks good and very well trimmed always looks the best.

CHIP Z'NUFF: No hair anywhere except on the head. Everything is much cleaner, easier to take care of and looks better. You can see what you're doing. I don't know anybody that has a ZZ Top beard down there. Back in the Seventies and the Eighties when I was a little kid I'm sure they had that, but nowadays I think people have grabbed on to the fact that it's better and cleaner; hygiene-wise it's much more manageable not having hair anywhere except on your head.

COURTNEY TAYLOR-TAYLOR: It depends on how much they naturally have. Like, a good Scandinavian Swede with just a cute little bush and very little on the undercarriage, naturally, that one is worth more than its weight in gold.

DANKO JONES: I'm one of those rare guys who likes it any which way the woman pleases, as long as it's not like a jungle. I like it completely shaved. I really like it shaved but there's the tuft throughout, like using the number one on the razor. And I don't mind it if the girl (if she's hot enough) wants to grow it out, then that's fine by me too. I don't care. I do not like it when girls get creative and if their name starts with S then they have an S down there. It just tells me that that person has a lot of time on their hands.

DOUG ROBB: I would say, at the most, maybe like a little landing strip. I don't know if that's a cultural thing. I don't mind no hair at all, but definitely not a Seventies bush.

EVAN SEINFELD: None, there should be none. If you have an excellent Beverly Hills waxer and you'd like to have a small Brazilian strip, make sure it's as narrow as your inner labia. Anything more than that makes you retro.

HANDSOME DICK MANITOBA: Minimal these days, minimal. A little spot here and there is OK. It's funny, like, pubic eras… This photographer Robert Bailey gave me a picture of The Dictators recently from CBGB's in 1976 and a girl had jumped on stage and pulled her pants down and you could tell it was the Seventies by her bush. I was like, 'That's a Seventies bush!' It's amazing how pubic hair has style. But for me these days, little or nothing is the best.

JAMES KOTTAK: Zero.

JESSE HUGHES: As much as they like but it depends what they're trying to turn on. If it's the get-the-fuck-out-of-here button, they might want to have a lot. If they're trying to turn on the stay-and-let's-hang-out button, they might want to do something totally different.

JIMMY ASHHURST: A very small amount. I'm excited to see that this custom is catching on globally. There was a time that it was only in more Westernised cities that you would find this idea of the trim. I used to think that completely shaved was the best, but I've seen some interesting works of art that can be done with a good pair of clippers these days. So I'm thinking the old racing strip is a pretty good turn-on.

LEMMY: I like a slight bush. It's not the most attractive part of a female's body, that's for sure. To me personally, a slight bush is good, but not an afro.

NICKE BORG: I'll be punished in hell for doing this interview with you… it very much depends on what kind of girl it is, but nobody really wants to bring scissors just to have sex. But it can also be a bit of a turn-off if it's like… [makes squeaky noises]. So, a nice little landing field is best.

ROB PATTERSON: Zero!

TOBY RAND: For me it would be none or a well cultivated area, like a strip or a triangular section.

VAZQUEZ: I want the full fucking disco bush, man. And I don't fucking care who thinks I'm an idiot – that is what I want. To me, it's like shaving your eyebrows off your face! You know what I'm saying? That would just look stupid. Keep it there man. It's got an aroma to it; it's got a feel to it. There are pheromones in that shit, man. I'm passionate about that; I'm real passionate about that.

What pubic hair maintenance should a guy perform?

ACEY SLADE: I didn't really realise until I was in a touring band that guys had to pay attention to hygiene. Until you're like changing in the hall of a bus – us rock'n'roll guys don't go to the gym or anything like that – so you're changing and you see stuff. I didn't realise that was so important and all of a sudden I started asking girls, 'So what do you think about grooming?' Apparently they like it. But I guess it depends on the person too. I was in a band with a keyboard player who made it a point to walk around in his underwear with his big man-bush sticking out either side of his tighty-whiteys and he'd swear the girls loved it. I don't get that. I was also in a band with a guy who shaved himself clean and I don't quite get that either.

ADDE: It shouldn't look like a forest when they go down there. Keep the hair out of the cock.

EVERYBODY'S DIFFERENT BUT GUYS CAN GET AWAY WITH MORE HAIR BECAUSE WOMEN AREN'T AS WEIRD.

ALLISON ROBERTSON: Everybody's different but guys can get away with more hair because women aren't as weird. I don't think women are as picky and women also like men to be manly, so it would be weird if they were always kind of bare. But I think if it's getting in the way of your girlfriend doing anything down there, you've got to trim. It goes both ways; it's the same for either.

ANDREW W.K.: I'd say between three and seven on the scale. Now, if you want to go down to zero, I would say that is a fun experience to have done it. To return to that early state reminds you of before you began to grow but it itches a lot, so I think once you do that once, you've got to maintain it I guess, otherwise it's really uncomfortable. It's exciting though. It's like, everyone should have a shaved head at one point in their life; I think everybody should shave themselves completely at one point.

BLASKO: Well, I keep it pretty fit and trim down there.

BRENT MUSCAT: I guess it just depends. I've always done different stuff. Sometimes I've been like the full Seventies bush, sometimes I shave it down bald. But I think the best thing is for guys to just be trimmed up a little bit. Just take it down an inch so there's hair there but it's not super long.

CHIP Z'NUFF: You'd better trim up too OK, because nobody wants to see a ZZ Top beard on a man either, so they've got to trim up and keep themselves together too. It's very important to show the girl that you care, and you care about yourself too. It's good for you.

COURTNEY TAYLOR-TAYLOR: It just depends: you don't want to be the Mr Shaved Bag or anything freaky or pervy gay-porn style. So I would actually say very little unless you're just a woolly mammoth with a nasty fucking thing that's oily, bristly and brutal.

DANKO JONES: It's got to be groomed too. The same as I want on a girl, I've got to be able to do the same thing. It's definitely a stickler for me – pubic hair maintenance, for sure.

DOUG ROBB: It's similar to ladies but don't go bald; that's not right. I would say just trim it, like with something you'd shave your head with and take it down to like a number one, so it's not like a giant afro.

EVAN SEINFELD: It depends if he's a guy in porn films or just a regular guy. For a regular guy, I don't think we should shave but we should trim; say a standard buzzer with a number one cut. Keep it short and out of the way.

HANDSOME DICK MANITOBA: Trimmed, I guess. I trim it. I think when it comes to the pubic region, care, and being a grown-up and taking care of your body and taking care of yourself is a turn-on.

JAMES KOTTAK: Keep it manscape. Manscape a bit. Keep it uniform.

JESSE HUGHES: Unless he's related to Sasquatch, he shouldn't really have to perform too much. I'm a ginger-haired boy and I'm Black Irish, so I'm blessed in all departments.

JIMMY ASHHURST: Keep it tight, keep it tight. You don't want to have the old piss diaper down there.

LEMMY: I always comb my pubic hairs to the left. Nah, I think shaving's the best. Chicks like that because they think it's clean.

NICKE BORG: It depends on what kind of girl you date and whether you want to look like her. I think that men and women – we have hair – fine. There was like a sudden trend that happened many years ago that people shave their balls, shave their whatever… Sometimes I'm like completely shaved; sometimes I don't give a flying shit. I once met a girl, and I didn't even have that much hair and she was like, 'Dude, you're hairy' and I'm like, 'Fuck you!' But sometimes I'll be like completely shaved and a girl will be like, 'Wow, you shave, you kinky bastard' and I'll be like, 'What?' So I think it's like a daily mood – it depends.

ROB PATTERSON: Zero!

TOBY RAND: Personally, I look after my ass and balls and that's about it. It gives me pleasure as well. It makes my dick look bigger too.

VAZQUEZ: Man, I'm like Burt Reynolds in 1977, man. I don't fucking maintain shit.

What's the best way to remove and maintain pubic hair?

BLASKO: For guys, on the sack you are going to want to get a razor and for on the upper portion, you get like body grooming clippers with a guard on.

ROB PATTERSON: Clippers if you're a guy; wax if a girl.

TOBY RAND: With your partner when you're having a bottle of red wine. You're pissed and you get the wax out and have a bit of fun with each other. That's the best way.

How frequently should one shower to be attractive to their partner?

ACEY SLADE: Oh, every day. If you're a female partner then definitely every day, but for guys, every couple of days.

ALLISON ROBERTSON: I shower every day, but I think some guys can get away with not showering maybe two days, three days. It all depends on how good you smell. I also think that some people are just attracted to each other with pheromones and stuff. Some people can handle how their partner's armpit smells. I think if you're really in love with somebody and are into somebody sexually, you actually don't care if they're kind of dirty. I tend to gravitate towards people who are somewhat more on the clean side.

BLASKO: You could probably get away with a day, a day-and-a-half, two days possibly, but whenever you go and do number two, you're going to have to take a shower at that point.

BRENT MUSCAT: Well I shower every day, so I think that's probably a pretty good start. If you shower in the morning and you go to work and you sweat all day, you should shower again at night. So I would say once a day, maybe up to twice a day if you need it, depending if you're a person who has body odour or sweats a lot.

CHIP Z'NUFF: Every day. Every day. Every single day you should be cleaned up, tidied up, because you don't know who you're going to run into. Be prepared at all times, gentlemen. That's what I think. You don't get a second chance on a first impression.

DANKO JONES: I shower once a day. Anything more than that, unless you're caught in a heat wave, I think is a little excessive, depending on what you do during the day. Sometimes I end up showering twice when I'm on tour just because there's a lot of sweat from the show, but other than that once a day.

EVAN SEINFELD: Oh showering, ladies, is an everyday event. Feel free to douche as well. We don't want any flavours. We don't need any Summer Musk, just plain-old unscented.

HANDSOME DICK MANITOBA: There can't be enough. If I don't know a girl and I pick up a girl the first time, it's like, 'We're going in the shower first. I'm going to clean that thing just in case you don't, and if you do, great, you'll be double-washed.' I'm a big fan of the totality of the sexual experience. There are many details in the total experience and smell is… I mean, if my nose gets near a girl's forearm and there's a smell I don't like, forget it! What am I going downstairs for? It's going to get worse. But I have friends who are like, 'The funkier the better.' There are different kinds of people in the world. Me, I can't throw them in the shower fast enough – and myself too. I want to know that wherever you go, with whatever part of your body you go with, it's going to smell pleasant and enjoyable. That's very important to me with both giving and taking.

JAMES KOTTAK: It depends but I guess at least once a week.

JESSE HUGHES: For me, I shower every day and I wash my hair every other day.

JIMMY ASHHURST: Oh God, daily, by all means. I used to think that there was an alternative to that but I've come to realise that's not the case. Two things to remember when living the touring lifestyle: bathe often, and keep moving.

LEMMY: Just before.

ROB PATTERSON: Never… just kidding. I like a little stink. Not too much though, so every other day maybe.

TOBY RAND: Well you'd be hoping once a day, but then again when you're on the road you don't really know do you? In my case, I'll shower when I want; I'm pretty clean.

VAZQUEZ: I tend to shower at least every other day. With girls, it's kind of different. With having long hair it's a pain in the ass to do every day, so I'd say every other day.

Is underarm odour a turn-on for your partner?

ACEY SLADE: Actually, I had a girl who used to like to huff my armpits. Swear to God, she would throw me down on the bed and stick her face in my armpits to smell them. I thought it was the funniest fucking thing in the world. I dated a girl from Germany one time and she had a little bit of armpit body odour and I was kind of weird with it. One day we were hanging out and she's putting her clothes back on and put on some men's deodorant. I was like, 'You wear men's deodorant?' and she was like, 'Yeah, you've probably noticed I've got really bad BO and I do everything I can do about it, so fuck it, what else can I do? So I wear guy's deodorant.' I thought that was so funny and so cool that it never bothered me again. It was like the pink elephant was out of the room now.

ADDE: The thing about smell is that if you find someone attractive you can even get attracted by their smell and their sweat. So it depends on the situation. I can get turned on by someone whose sweat I can smell, but if I'm not turned on I think it's the most disgusting smell ever.

ANDREW W.K.: I don't know but certainly being able to smell the natural aroma of somebody – odour is normally a bad word but aroma is usually a good word – the oils, people have a certain smell. Covering that up with perfume or deodorant is one thing to do. Using perfume to mix with your natural smell is also another, but I don't know that smelling bad is ever a turn-on to anybody. I guess there's probably people out there, but not to me.

BLASKO: I know that it is for some people. I know that it can be.

BRENT MUSCAT: I don't mind if you can smell them a little bit, as long as they don't stink. Everybody has a natural smell to their body I guess, or some kind of body odour, and as long as it's not pungent I think it's fine. A tiny bit is OK but depending on the extent of your body odour… I use underarm deodorant every day. I take a shower every day and I use cologne when I go out at night to a club, so I try to smell good all the time. I think girls do too, but depending on the girl, if they have a problem, there's things they could do like use deodorant, or they could wash, or use different products.

COURTNEY TAYLOR-TAYLOR: Only for sociopathic art school students.

DANKO JONES: Not for me man, it's a turn-off.

DOUG ROBB: If it is, I haven't been told that. I've been told, 'Man, your shit stinks' before.

EVAN SEINFELD: A lot of European girls like to have it and smell it and I understand the pheromone attraction but you know what; I'm a shallow American guy. Ladies, no hair and no odour, we're good.

JAMES KOTTAK: No! It's a turn-off! Buy some deodorant.

JIMMY ASHHURST: I think not. Although it's a big planet and there are a lot of people on it. I'm sure you'll find there's someone into just about anything you can imagine and some things you shouldn't. I'm sure there are some people who are into guitar techs with spina bifida as well.

NICKE BORG: No, c'mon. Like, some people use showers; some people don't. And I hate someone who's fucking overdone with fucking aftershave, whatever perfume. The best thing is like totally natural – I just had a shower and this is the way I smell – fine. And then you get sweaty when you have sex or whatever and then a little bit of that smell of being sweaty… it's fucking awesome.

ROB PATTERSON: Absolutely!

TOBY RAND: It's a bit of a turn-off for me, but then again if the girl is hot and she's fucking awesome, it doesn't really matter.

VAZQUEZ: I actually really like that. Maybe I'm the first one to answer yes on this one but the thing is man, it's like so awesome when you're just fucking a girl and you get your face into her armpit and you can smell that – it's crazy. My theory is that thousands of years ago when people didn't go to a movie together on a date, or they couldn't have a favourite song together, I think a lot of people's chemistry was based on could they stand each other's smell. So I think it's some sort of ancient fucking thing man – there's something chemical going on there and it's fucking hot.

What's the worst smelling vagina you've encountered?

ACEY SLADE: It was in New Orleans. This should have been a clue from the get-go: we played this show and I got hit with the keyboard and got a gash down the side of my head with stitches, so I had this big fucking wound on the side of my head. I'd met this stripper in a strip bar on Bourbon St earlier. So she comes to the show. She has a place and we go back to her flat and it's the coolest flat in the world. New Orleans is like my favourite place. Literally, when I got her naked, before much foreplay, the room stunk so badly! I had every intention of staying at this amazing flat. I got there and I was like, 'Fuck yeah man, I'm crashing here, taking a shower.' She was really pretty but she smelled so bad, as soon as I got done, I ran! I would have run sooner if I wasn't already naked.

ADDE: Oh this Yugoslavian woman… I came down to her belly button area when we were taking a bath and I could feel this awful smell. I was like, 'I'm not going to go down there.' I wasn't even going to kiss her belly… and we were in a bath! We washed, but it didn't help. That was one of the worst fucking smells I've ever experienced!

ANDREW W.K.: Oh geez! Well, one of my earlier girlfriends definitely had some hygiene issues. I guess because she was just so young and no one had ever told her or taught her about that and I didn't really know what it was caused by either, but I guess yeast infections or other infections or issues with bacteria really created the smelly situations in my earlier years. It can be very traumatising because it took a long time before I realised that's not how a girl always is. That something's very wrong when there's a smell like that.

CHIP Z'NUFF: I've been pretty lucky; I've got to be honest with you. I haven't been with anything that terrible. I've been lucky. I haven't experienced anything difficult. My friends tell me they always do the test just to make sure: touch down with their fingers and the old sniffy-poo on the nose. I know it sounds adolescent, but it's tried and true. It's been working for hundreds of years. But things have changed now and the brochure's out. Keep it clean and keep yourself together if you're going to have any action, so I think most people know about that. At least they do in this country.

COURTNEY TAYLOR-TAYLOR: Oh fuck, that is funny. Um, man. Also pretty much half a football field of lawn was on that one too. Like, surprise, I've got a pelt, an entire pelt. A little further and I'd be digging around to find her navel. Ironically, years and years and years and years later, a friend of mine divorced from his wife and he was just kind of depressed (he's a studio engineer and just a fucking genius), so I said come on tour with us and do live sound. We were having a ball on tour and one night we were drunk and he said, 'We've crossed paths before.' I'm like, 'What is that innuendo? What is that code for?' and he's like, 'Same girl.' I'm like, 'We fucking grew up in Portland, Oregon, dude. There was like nine. Are you fucking kidding me? You only know about one? Which one?' He told me and I was like, 'Man, I didn't touch it! Are you kidding? That was the stinkiest!' He's like, 'Oh my God! That's so weird! That was the stinkiest, blah blah blah.'

Apparently, he had gone out with this girl for a number of months and she was a really good girl, so he kind of fell in love with her. For me, it was only a matter of a couple of dates, but it stopped pretty much right there for him too. Being young and in your early twenties, you don't really know how to tell them about that. For me, it was just a sort of a dirty, poo thing, but apparently he went ahead and told her and abruptly disappeared. Ironically, my worst as it would be was somebody else's worst too, but it was somebody I know. Furthermore on that matter, let me tell you how you tell somebody: you act real surprised and concerned and you go, 'Honey, I think there's something wrong here. This doesn't smell right. Honey, are you OK?' like you're concerned. You're not grossed out, you're not freaked out, you are concerned. 'You get could very ill. You might be ill, are you OK?' You're a wonderful and caring man.

SHE WAS REALLY PRETTY BUT SHE SMELLED SO BAD, AS SOON AS I GOT DONE, I RAN! I WOULD HAVE RUN SOONER IF I WASN'T ALREADY NAKED.

DANKO JONES: It's absolutely horrid! It is like the worst meal gone bad. It is just the worst. It's like a fish store that's been closed down for two weeks. It's fucking bad! It's really fucking bad!

DOUG ROBB: Probably my first girlfriend ever. It has nothing to do with rock'n'roll or whatever, but it does have a lot to do with being 16 or 17 and not knowing any better.

GINGER: I used to date a girl with what I can only assume was a yeast infection. She'd get out of the bath and still smell bad. I later found out that she wasn't the entirely faithful type, so it makes sense she'd smell a bit used.

HANDSOME DICK MANITOBA: Yeah, forget it. You've got to send a scout down; I'm not that brave. I've had situations where I'm like, 'You know what? I don't feel so good' or something. It's not an obligation; it's supposed to be a pleasure.

JIMMY ASHHURST: There's nothing quite like that odour. I have an imprint of it on my mind and if I tend to think about it too much it comes back to me, so we should move on to the next question.

LEMMY: I don't know really. What, you want the name?

NICKE BORG: I was once with a girl who did not shave and obviously I don't think she had a shower either for the last few days and it was very horrible. That kind of smell is something you don't really want to recall in a way. I can't describe how it smelled… very, very, pfff, wow, yuk.

ROB PATTERSON: Ewww... No comment.

TOBY RAND: You know when you drive behind a garbage truck? Like seriously! When there's just a mass of pubic hair and you realise you've just been playing a festival for four days and it's the last night and you realise everyone's been camping and there's no real access to showers. That is the equivalent of smelling like a garbage truck and my worst experience of smells yet.

VAZQUEZ: I remember a long time ago I slept with this girl and I was going to go down on her and she was like, 'Oh no, don't.' So I was like OK whatever, I just fucked her instead. I was going to take the condom off after it's all done and my fingers got wet when I took the condom off. I kind of like smelled my fingers man and I was like, 'Jesus fucking Christ, man!' It smelled like dirty fucking dishes or something.

KISSING & CARESSING

"COVER HER BREASTS IN CHAMPAGNE THEN LICK-FLICK AND SUCK OFF EVERY LAST DROP. SHE GETS AROUSED WHILE YOU GET TO DRINK"

What's the best way to instigate a kiss?

ACEY SLADE: I think to grab a girl gently by the back of the hair, not in a mean way, but to let her know you're going to give her a kiss.

ADDE: Just flatter them as much as possible. It's important for eye contact when it comes to a woman – it's important.

ALLISON ROBERTSON: If I start the kiss, then I usually go for the cheek and move their head. I can be kind of aggressive, so that's usually what I do. You get to know somebody, you're talking, you're flirting, and if you feel like it's about time to make a move and they're not doing it, I just move in really close and kiss on the cheek first.

ANDREW W.K.: I don't think there's anything wrong with asking or saying that you'd like to kiss the other person. Maybe that makes it more awkward in a way, so use your judgement. The word kiss is a really nice word. Gene Simmons and Paul Stanley and their advisors understood that. It comes off the tongue nicely and I think it's a great way to do it. It's memorable and it's respectful and it's gentle. Otherwise, leaning in and going for it as it always happens in the movies, but I never really remembered it happening like that to me. It was always a little more awkward and that's what made it kind of exciting.

BRENT MUSCAT: I think if you're with someone on a date and there's maybe like a dark area and if they're looking at you and you're looking in their eyes, I think you should just make the move. Just kind of go for it; maybe not crazy-like, but a small one at least first of all. Maybe even a kiss on the cheek to start and see the reaction you get. Even with that, at least it's a start.

CHIP Z'NUFF: Doing something nice for somebody. I wouldn't go making out right away too. A nice conversation and something that's said that's funny or charming. That's a tough question, to be honest with you. You just know by instinct! You can just tell by instinct. If you're a guy and you're not sure about it, when she goes to give you a kiss goodbye or a kiss on the cheek for something, turn real quick and kiss her on the mouth. That seems to work pretty good without being embarrassing. You both laugh about it and that might get the ball rolling for a second kiss.

COURTNEY TAYLOR-TAYLOR: Ask.

DANKO JONES: Just lean forward I guess. You kind of instinctually know the moment I think.

DOUG ROBB: That's more of a feel thing. If you think she might want to kiss you, you should just go for it.

EVAN SEINFELD: If you are trying to coax a girl into kissing you I would say touch her face; I would think touch her face and make eye contact. She'll give you a green light or not at that point, but understand it's the lady's choice.

HANDSOME DICK MANITOBA: You're asking for details of something that just happens. Like, I have to rewind the tape, but I think it is body language and eyes. I always think you should stay in the moment and don't be so neurotic about your own behaviour and your own nervousness, or your own self-consciousness let's say. Don't make it about you; start off by being in the moment and read the body language, read the girl's eyes. Look in her eyes. She'll kind of let you know through her body language and eye contact whether it's OK to come closer. And once you're at a certain body language angle and you're talking... I think you talk with the eyes first, then the lips. Then at some point, without being too aggressive about it, you have to plant a small kiss or something to say, 'I'm making my move. I'm a man and I'm taking control of this situation.' You have to take that little leap of faith at some point based on eyes and body language, and then you go for it, knowing that the worst that can happen is you get a no, or you get a yes. That might be the most exciting moment of courtship, jumping that little bridge, making that move.

JAMES KOTTAK: Say, 'Kiss me.'

JESSE HUGHES: Put your lips on another or just say, 'Can I kiss you?' or walk out of the bathroom completely naked with an erection. That's the best way to engineer a kiss!

JIMMY ASHHURST: Timing is everything man. Mid-drink or mid-conversation is normally not the best time to do it. Or with a mouthful of catering is probably not a good idea either. So I think timing is everything; if you can find the moment, you're going to get kissed back.

JOEL O'KEEFFE: Drop something that falls down next to them, so when you lean in to pick it up your lips come so close that you may as well give them a kiss on the way down.

LEMMY: Usually, placing the lips together is good; hers and yours. I don't know of any other way of doing it really.

NICKE BORG: I think that when you accidentally just move closer and closer to each other without even thinking about it and all of a sudden you're just there – lip to lip. It's like, you're talking and moving slowly, slowly, closer and closer, then bang – your lips are sealed! Then if your kiss after that is fucking great, you're caught.

ROB PATTERSON: Grab the motherfucking back of the head by the hair.

TOBY RAND: I like to go for the side of their neck first, before I touch their lips. That way you get the feeling and the vibe for it. I think the anticipation of a kiss is always the most fun as well. If you ask me and my friends, the excitement of the almost kiss is one of the best feelings you'll ever have. So I like to play around the lips before I get to them.

I LIKE TO GO FOR THE SIDE OF THEIR NECK FIRST, BEFORE I TOUCH THEIR LIPS. THAT WAY YOU GET THE FEELING AND THE VIBE FOR IT.

VAZQUEZ: I'm just so full of myself and I'm so fucking confident that I'm just going to go for it. I'm just going to pull her close and that's it. You know what? It works every time.

How do you make a kiss memorable?

ADDE: Give her tongue like a blowjob. That's what I would do.

ALLISON ROBERTSON: I read something once and you know what? It works. This isn't necessarily making it memorable, but instead of trying to make your mark and do something weird, like bite someone and hurt them or do something they don't necessarily like, what I read (and I've noticed it works) is you try and see how the other person kisses and then you kind of try and mirror it. Not like trying to do exactly what they want, you have to incorporate what you both want, but I feel like when you try to get to know whatever they're doing and match it up a little, then that's how they remember it.

ANDREW W.K.: It seems like the location of where you are when it happens. Are you still out in public, are you back in someone's house, are you kind of away around a corner? Like in a bar, you go in the back by the phone booth or something. I think it depends on where you were when you remember back to your first kiss.

BRENT MUSCAT: If you're at a cool dating spot, like a nice hotel or at the beach as a memorable spot, I think the kiss is going to be memorable too.

COURTNEY TAYLOR-TAYLOR: Dry, soft and sweet as pie. That's how I would, anyway.

DANKO JONES: Just be a good kisser, I guess.

DOUG ROBB: I don't know man. I think they either are or they aren't. You can't be like, 'Watch this! I'm going to do a memorable kiss on this one. I'm going to do a forgetful one on that one.'

EVAN SEINFELD: To make a kiss memorable you squeeze her ass really hard.

GINGER: Kissing is so personal that it's impossible to answer that one objectively. I think it's really important to find a chemistry in kissing, and allow each other a little time to get to know how their new partner likes to be kissed. If kissing is a battle of wills then the relationship will suffer the same fate.

HANDSOME DICK MANITOBA: There's no rule of thumb for them. I think it's like the magic of life, the magic of connecting and it just happens.

JAMES KOTTAK: Say, 'Don't forget this kiss!'

JESSE HUGHES: By having the biggest boner in the world while you're kissing her.

JIMMY ASHHURST: You've got to work with the other person. The first one is usually a bit of an exploration and can be a little odd but as you start to get to know the person... That's the most fun in getting to know someone; figuring that stuff out; how best you work together.

JOEL O'KEEFFE: Put your heart and everything into it... and her!

LEMMY: Let off a firecracker while you're kissing her. Or if your head blows up; that's always good.

ROB PATTERSON: Do it when they are not expecting it!

TOBY RAND: By putting everything into it first time and making sure that you look into their eyes when you're doing it.

VAZQUEZ: If it's with me then it should be memorable.

What's a good turn-on move to do when kissing?

ACEY SLADE: I'm a big hair-puller. What can I say? Maybe that's my fetish?

ALLISON ROBERTSON: It depends on where you are but I like grabbing people's heads and stuff. Some guys don't like their hair touched or whatever, but I like touching their head. Not necessarily pulling their hair, but kind of rubbing their head or their neck. And I also think, for me, I like it when guys hold you. It's kind of weird when they're afraid to touch. You feel like you want to be able to relax and feel like you're in a little bit of a grip. I like that.

JAMES KOTTAK: The old rubbing the neck thing works.

JIMMY ASHHURST: The old hand around the back of the neck is usually a good one for me. Maybe that goes back to the bondage question; I'm not sure.

JOEL O'KEEFFE: With one hand grabbing the booty, unclip her bra with the other. Or for something a little more gutsy, drop a couple of digits in the wonder down under and get busy with the frizzy!

ROB PATTERSON: That's secret.

TOBY RAND: Sucking the bottom lip really hard, really hard, and once again looking them in the eyes while you're doing it. If a girl does that to me it's like, 'Holy shit! You're awesome.'

VAZQUEZ: Maybe this makes me look creepy but in my mind it turns them on: when I'm making out with a girl I like to take my hand and like slide my fingers down the small of her back so my fingers are just like in her ass crack. I'm not a gentleman at all. I love public displays of affection.

Is there a way to fondle a breast to quickly arouse a woman?

ACEY SLADE: Inside the bra is a good help. That being said, nothing is a bigger turn-off than padded bras. I'd rather see a girl who's confident in her body. Most girls who don't have a big chest are probably pretty thin anyway. Nothing's worse than when you put a hand on a big padded bra.

ADDE: It's so different... some like it hard and some go 'Ouch', as some have sensitive nipples. So, you've just got to really feel what she's feeling.

ALLISON ROBERTSON: No. I think that all girls are different. Some girls like things really gentle, some girls like their boobs squeezed and I think there isn't necessarily a complete right way at all. I also think that even one girl will have a different reaction depending on who the guy is, whether or not they have good hands or weird hands. It completely doesn't matter. I think it depends.

BLASKO: I think anything like that you have to ease into with a woman. You don't want to jump right in, sticking your fingers in, or slapping them around, pinching and twisting. You've kind of got to like work your way up to that. Start out slow and work your way up to that.

BRENT MUSCAT: I wouldn't say too rough. I would say just to cup it and squeeze a little bit, gently kind of rub. Depending on the girl, I know sometimes girls' breasts get sore around their period so that may not be a great time to do it, so I think timing has to be right. Like I said, depending on the time of the month, the girl's breasts could be tender so start off slow and just see what kind of reaction you get. A lot of it is feedback; you do something and see what kind of reaction you get back, so it's like action/reaction. Starting out slow with anything is always the best move, and work your way up. If they like it, you can go a little bit more. If they moan a little with pleasure, you can turn it up a notch at a time. If they're getting into it, you can ask them, 'Hey how's that? What do you like?' If you get intimate with someone and you feel comfortable, you can always ask for feedback.

CHIP Z'NUFF: It depends what situation and where you're at with foreplay. Be gentle and nice with the nipples; kiss them softly, a little rubbing on them but not too hard. Don't be a jag-off and be selfish and hurt them. Be very gentle and nice, then once the ball is rolling and there's action going on, then you can get a bit rougher, but in the beginning nice and soft is essential.

DANKO JONES: I've always noticed nipple play is good. Very manageable nipple play, just like not hard and not too soft usually works.

JAMES KOTTAK: I'm sure there is; I'm not the guy to ask.

JIMMY ASHHURST: A real one or a fake one? I understand there's not as much feeling in the fake ones. It all depends on being able to read the girl and listen to noises – that's usually a good indicator of what's working and what isn't.

JOEL O'KEEFFE: Cover her breasts in champagne then lick-flick and suck off every last drop. She gets aroused while you get to drink.

LEMMY: You should go around the nipple, not pinch it or bite it or anything like that. You can spend three quarters of an hour biting the fucking thing, but if you run your finger around it about four times, you'll find the chick is much more teased by that.

NICKE BORG: I think just fucking leave them alone until she really wants you to touch her breasts. Just leave them alone; act like you don't even pay them attention – even if they're big, small, great, whatever – so she'll be like, 'What the fuck? He doesn't want to touch my tits' and *then* you do it.

ROB PATTERSON: Just don't be hard. Women like everything soft, to a point.

TOBY RAND: Grab the breast full and massage it, like you'd massage anything, and then play with the nipple like you're playing with a spinning top… but not flicking too hard. It never goes astray to lick your finger and do it, if you're in the mood.

VAZQUEZ: That depends on the woman: some women have really sensitive nipples and I've met girls who can have an orgasm from playing with their nipples. And I've met girls who are like, 'Do not touch my nipples or I'll punch you in the face because it hurts.' With some women, it just doesn't do anything, so it goes back to the whole thing about asking them.

What places on the body can be caressed to turn on a partner most?

BLASKO: All places really. I don't really feel there's any limits, unless of course they're ticklish, then there's an issue. Anywhere is fair game.

DANKO JONES: I call it the shelf, which is the curve of a woman's back from the bottom of her back to the ass. I really like women who have nice shelves, meaning it's almost an L-shape or a C-shape on their back. Usually it comes from dancing when they're little girls, like ballet when they're little girls, and they usually get the nice curve. So that area, plus the back of the neck and the licking of arms sometimes.

JOEL O'KEEFFE: That truly depends on the girl but like I said before, her body is a temple and her pussy is the front door, so make sure you make a big entrance and she'll *always* want you coming back for more.

ROB PATTERSON: Hmm… anywhere, if done right.

TOBY RAND: I love to grab a girl on her lower ass, in between her thigh and her ass, and just kind of lift her off the ground a bit. That always seems to add a bit of excitement after that.

MARRIAGE

"IF YOU OPEN HER CAR DOOR ON THE PASSENGER SIDE AND LET HER IN, IF SHE LEANS OVER TO UNLOCK YOUR DOOR ON THE DRIVER'S SIDE, SHE'S THE ONE"

How do you raise the issue of a pre-nuptial agreement?

ALLISON ROBERTSON: I think it makes sense to have one, depending on how much money is involved, or if one makes more money than the other. I think that you have to bring that up before you even get engaged, or right when you get engaged.

DANKO JONES: You just do. It's a topic of discussion that should be easily brought up if you two are very open and honest and know each other. It shouldn't be an issue.

DOUG ROBB: I would say if you're going to go that route, you have to be upfront with it pretty early on in a relationship. If you're marrying someone (hopefully it doesn't happen in two weeks) and if you're in a relationship, after a while it's bound to come up. Probably around the same time marriage comes up if you're dating somebody. When it comes up, if that's what you want to do, you've just got to be honest and say, 'That's how I feel. That's what I want to do. If we ever need to get to that point, you know where I stand and I know where you stand' and take it from there. It's definitely not something you want to spring last moment, like the day before the wedding or something.

EVAN SEINFELD: If you're starting to feel serious about a girl you should start telling stories about happy marriages involving pre-nups and how much women who are confident enough at the end of the road don't have to suck a man dry. Refer to women without pre-nuptials as vampires, parasites and vultures. Kind of, don't give the woman a choice whether to agree or not.

JAMES KOTTAK: You hire a lawyer for that one. Forget it for divorce, but you definitely hire a lawyer for that one.

JESSE HUGHES: You don't.

ROB PATTERSON: You just do it. There's no question about that.

When do you know it's time to marry the one you are with?

ACEY SLADE: From my experience, that's kind of tough. For me, I was a 34-year-old rock'n'roll guy who'd been sowing his wild oats for years. When I did get married, I had a lot of red flags and a lot of signs that maybe I should wait on this. That whole thing got played back on me like, 'You're this rock'n'roll guy who's never going to commit. How am I supposed to have any security?' Trust your gut on it. I guess that's really the bottom line. I had that whole role reversal thing like, 'You're only nervous because you're never going to make a commitment.' Well, I thought it, so maybe that's true, maybe that's right? My gut was right, so stick with your gut.

ADDE: When she turns you on and accepts you for being on the road, like *every* day of the year.

ALLISON ROBERTSON: I don't think it's even necessarily 'time to marry': I've been married but it wasn't my idea and I went along with it because it seemed like the right thing to do. But as far as I can tell, to me marriage is more like if you're going to have kids and it just starts to make more sense to be married than to not be married, in that kind of a thing. Otherwise, I think there is no 'time' to get married. I don't think you have to be married. I think you can either trust somebody or you can't. You can live with someone or you can't, and you want to be with somebody forever or you don't. I feel like being married doesn't make any of the problems go away. People still cheat, or not. Fuck it, it doesn't matter.

ANDREW W.K.: I've only been married once and, for me, it was a feeling of when you're no longer looking at your girlfriend as a girlfriend. It's when you don't have a concept of them that relates to all the other girls or relationships you've ever been in. When you realise that the space they occupy isn't that of a girl or a woman or a person, but as your partner. It's a very intense feeling and you can tell it when you can tell it; you can tell that this is the person you can imagine being with forever and if you can't imagine that, I don't think you should do it. You have to be able to fathom that and even though that's really impossible to picture because you can't really experience all that in one thought, you should be able to picture the circumstances as they are now being forever. Meaning, the way that person exists, exists like my Mum or my Dad or my brother. They're a primary, elemental idea; they exist in a state that is as singular as myself and not as one in a series or an idea of someone, but as someone who is as important as I am.

BLASKO: I think you just kind of know. At some point, you're like, 'Hey this just feels right', you know? 'Let's go for it!'

BRENT MUSCAT: There's that old saying that you just know. I didn't know that until I found the one and when I found it, I just knew it. It's really like that. You have a feeling and you look at them and go, 'I don't want to be without her. This girl is everything I could see in my life.' You just know. You feel like they're smart enough, they make you a better person and add to you as a person, and they're definitely a good partner. I really do believe that you just kind of know. When you know it's the right one, you start really thinking about it too. You start thinking, 'I'd like to marry this woman.' You also feel that you don't want to lose them.

CHIP Z'NUFF: When she's pregnant. That's one way. If you're from a family like I am, you don't have a baby out of wedlock. But: time. Time is the essence, right there. If you're spending quality time with someone, you'll know. You'll know right away, but wait a few years for sure before you jump into that fucking deep water, just to make sure. My recommendation would be to live together for a while. I recommend if you really love somebody and they love you, move in and live together and see how it goes. Make sure you pay your bills and stuff and don't be hitting the fucking strip clubs and bars every fucking night with your friends. If you love her and you want to spend time with her, that's the woman of the future for you, that's what I would do. I've been married 23 years; 15 to my first wife, eight to my second, so I do know how it works and that's the best advice I can give anybody: don't get married right away, move in first.

COURTNEY TAYLOR-TAYLOR: When about five years has elapsed. When you have gone so long, so many years, five years, having only one meltdown a year, no more, and you're still amazed with this person. So amazed with them that they're still, in your mind, a better person, that you have to be on your best behaviour and watch it all the time in order to keep them. Right? Because then you know that you are really that person and you can be that strong and comfortable and patient and interesting and fun and sexy. You're going to know that about yourself, which is killer to know that you really are a great boyfriend; a real honey to have. You also know that they could not have faked it for that long either without that truly being a part of their personality and their make-up and probably just trying to live up to your idea of them too. But guess what? If they can do it for five fucking years, they are it!

DANKO JONES: When you have no interest in anybody else, serious interest in anybody else and you don't foresee there are any other options. A lot of people are in relationships, but the reason they push back when push comes to shove is because in the back of their heads, whether they're going to admit it or not, they're waiting for something better to come along. When that idea or that option is erased, then you can marry that person.

DOUG ROBB: I don't want to use the cop-out of answering, 'Well, you just know.' I think there's a lot that goes into it. If you're lucky enough, you'll meet lots of people in your life and share experiences and have relationships. In the case with me, there was always that one, for reasons too many to list, that always had it coming. And I kind of think that goes into it; just knowing that they're the one.

EVAN SEINFELD: When I saw my wife it was love at first sight. The first time I got married I knew it was a failure as I was doing it.

JAMES KOTTAK: If you open her car door on the passenger side and let her in, if she leans over to unlock your door on the driver's side, she's the one.

JESSE HUGHES: When you can see that the possibility of living comfortably with a person for the rest of your life and being committed to them. Then it's time; then there are no other questions. Everything else is immaterial. People spend a lot of time begging the question instead of answering it.

JIMMY ASHHURST: I will let you know; I don't have any idea.

I RECOMMEND IF YOU REALLY LOVE SOMEBODY AND THEY LOVE YOU, MOVE IN AND LIVE TOGETHER AND SEE HOW IT GOES.

NICKE BORG: Marriage is something that's been built up in modern times and, in a way, people are just pissing on it. They're like flushing it down the drain – get a marriage, get a divorce, get a marriage, get a divorce – like it's just something fun to do like having a fucking pint or something. No! Not being Christian or anything, but I was brought up in a small city with really religious parents where if you're going to get married, it's because you love that person so much and you want to make that commitment of like, 'I'm yours forever.' Really, it's just signing a paper, but there's something beautiful about it.

ROB PATTERSON: When you realise you can't live without them.

VAZQUEZ: When you know that they're there for you. They love you for you and they don't love you for who you are. It's almost better if they're not a fan. Let's face it – you're not always going to be that guy. Right now the business is all going to shit anyway, so it's not like any of us have any fucking money. You want to have someone that kind of understands the reality of what's really going on, instead of what they imagine it's like.

Is there an ideal way to propose?

ACEY SLADE: I think it should be unique; come up with something original. I was thinking of doing it atop the Empire State Building. That's cool but kind of a cliché.

ADDE: Down on your knees – get down on your knees and just ask her.

ALLISON ROBERTSON: No. I'm not that kind of girl that has some fantasy, but I do think that if you're going to propose it doesn't have to be original but it should be something that has a good memory attached to it. So I think a good way is like a traditional way or a way that is not going to be… I wouldn't want to be proposed to somewhere really depressing or like, 'Hey, you wanna marry me?' I feel that if someone's going to propose it should be a little bit more grandiose, not necessarily at a dinner or whatever like in the movies, but definitely somewhere interesting or somewhere memorable.

ANDREW W.K.: I think making it more formal and more intense is better. Same way when you have a wedding ceremony, I think having a large ceremony with a lot of people and doing it very traditionally has value and I never would have thought that before. Before I got married, a very wise friend of mine who had been married before and was much older than me told me that when he gets married again he's going to have a much more formal ceremony. I said, 'Why?' and he said, 'Well our first ceremony we did it really funny. It was really low-key, we had it on the beach, there was all kinds of people dressed crazy, we didn't have a lot of our family there and the marriage was terrible.' He thinks that they weren't taking it seriously enough to realise what they were getting into and the ceremony itself did reflect on that. So I think when you ask someone to marry you, have the ring (you don't necessarily have to get down on one knee) and plan on doing it. I don't think it should result out of a conversation. I don't know if you've seen the movie *Sex And The City*; remember that marriage proposal? That's probably the other end of the spectrum; a conversational agreement, but to each their own. I think that the more intense you can make the idea of what you're doing, the more aware you'll be of the implications.

BLASKO: I think girls like to have some kind of sense of tradition involved in it. Look, everyone's all for doing something creative, but I think the bare bones basic… you can't go wrong with getting on one knee, so long as you've got a ring. And talking to the dad is probably a good way to go first, too.

BRENT MUSCAT: It's funny, my wife always gives me a hard time because she's like, 'You never proposed to me!' I think it would have been nice if we did, but when we were thinking about getting married it was almost like we just talked about it together. My wife was from another country and she couldn't stay long in America and she was saying her parents were pressuring her to get married. They were sending her on dates to meet guys and stuff; they were being matchmakers while I was dating her! She even told me, 'Look, eventually I'm going to have to go back home' and we just talked about it. So I never actually proposed to her – so I wouldn't know. If I could go back in time, maybe I would do it, but I think at the time I was just so scared. I really thought that she was just too good for me and I was too scared she would say no, so we just talked about it and both agreed and both did it.

CHIP Z'NUFF: There are quite a few ways I would think. For me it was real simple. My first wife was my childhood sweetheart and after years and years of being together I just told her, 'We should be together forever', even though at the time I didn't know I was a liar. When you first get married you want it to be forever. You don't gear it up for failure. However, after a time you find yourself looking at the menu, even if not ordering you've still got to look around because we're men, we're animals. But if it's something really special and you really feel it, just let them know. Be honest. It's always good to be honest with the women. Let them know your feelings without being too sappy. Be a man about it.

COURTNEY TAYLOR-TAYLOR: Well if there is, I didn't do it.

DANKO JONES: I think getting on one knee is kind of hokey. I think the element of surprise is always fun and memorable.

DOUG ROBB: No, I don't think so. For a long time, I thought I was going to propose on stage in front of thousands of people. I thought about it, thinking it'll be cool and unique and all that kind of stuff. I ended up proposing to my wife in bed. I kind of got caught in a lie so I had to propose. I had been at her parents' house all day talking with her parents, basically asking for permission – the old-fashioned permission. She had been texting and calling me all day and I didn't answer the phone because I was at her parents' house. So I get home; she was bartending at the time and she gets home really late and I make up some cockamamie story like I forgot my phone at the studio and yadda yadda yadda. So she gets into bed and was like, 'So where were you today?' At that moment, I could either tell her what the fuck I was doing or by tomorrow her brother, who saw me at her parents' house, is going to say something like, 'Hey why was Doug over at your parents' house?' So I was like, 'Fuck it; I've got to just do it right now.' So I rolled over and wiped the boogers from my eyes and asked her to marry me at four in the morning in bed. The best part about it was I was wearing a T-shirt that my Dad had given me 12 years ago (or something like that) that he drew of me singing and underneath it says Doug of Hoobastank. So I was wearing a T-shirt of myself, which is pretty ridiculous, and asking my girl to marry me at four in the morning. So it was definitely not proposing in front of a stadium, but it was spontaneous and honest.

EVAN SEINFELD: I'm a hopeless romantic. I know I sound like a horrible pervert sometimes, but with my wife I got every cent I could together and I bought the biggest, best diamond I could find, and I put it in a gorgeous antique princess cut setting. I got down on one knee – actually in the middle of sex: I had this ring Federal Expressed to my hotel in South Beach, Miami and I got down on one knee. I think you can be cute and clever and have it come up on the JumboTron at the baseball game or something, but I think it's something you want to remember forever if it's someone you want to spend the rest of your life with.

GINGER: Privately and somewhere that you will both remember fondly as the place where it happened. Somewhere she loves.

JAMES KOTTAK: Any time, anywhere, whatever feels right.

JESSE HUGHES: The ideal way to propose is you pay the father of the bride 40,000 camels... No, I'm just kidding. The best way to propose, for me, is down on one knee.

JIMMY ASHHURST: I expect timing would be everything. Hopefully it would be a voluntary thing and not like, 'Oh hey, the DNA test is back and it's yours.' I think if it's voluntary on both sides then at least you're ahead of the game.

ROB PATTERSON: With a black diamond ring, on your knees.

VAZQUEZ: As long as you're not doing it at a bar, I think you're going to be OK. I think any woman, when you ask that question, they're going to be happy that you're doing it. I don't think they want you to make it a production, but it should definitely not be at the pub.

What would be a perfect marriage ceremony?

ACEY SLADE: I'll tell you what I did and I think it was perfect; I think it was ideal: we didn't have a lot of money and it was one of these things where she's from Denmark and I'm from here [USA], so how do we get everybody together? It got really complicated. The idea that I came up with was to volunteer as a helper in the New York City Halloween Parade. I called up the Halloween Parade people and said, 'What do you guys think of a couple getting married in the middle of the Halloween Parade?' and they said they thought it was the coolest idea they'd ever heard of. Even though we only had two dozen people who could attend the wedding because of the logistics of it, we did it in front of eight million people: there's four million in the parade and we did it on TV, which is another four million. So everyone was in costume, but the funniest part was that it seemed like a trick or treat thing but it was a real minister.

ADDE: One thing's for sure, I want *all* my friends there; all my friends to witness it and then it doesn't matter. It has to be a nice place, but the most ideal is to have all our friends there.

ALLISON ROBERTSON: It's hard to know. My parents are divorced but I always thought they had a really cool wedding. It was in the backyard. I was already born; they got married after they had me. I was a baby. It just seemed like a party with a lot of rock'n'rollers. My Dad was a musician and my Mum worked at a record label. And to me that is like the ultimate wedding ceremony: a lot more relaxed, non-denominational, no church, wearing whatever the hell you guys want. I think it's cool if the guy wears a weird suit (as long as it's not completely terrible or tragic) and the woman wears something that just expresses her style. I'm a fan of that. I've been to a lot of weddings of friends where it's traditional and it's cool but you've just stuck yourself into the cookie-cutter thing. I think it's much more interesting if you have a cool band play, or your friend's band play, or even just a terrible cover band and laugh hysterically at that. Good food. I just think it's good to customise it. I think it's so boring to do the normal thing.

BLASKO: I just went to Vegas and that was pretty perfect for me.

BRENT MUSCAT: Well I did three. I did one in America. It was great. It was April, so spring time. My uncle has a house in South Pasadena, which is a really beautiful area of South California and his backyard had all the flowers blooming and a really long, rectangular strip of grass surrounded by flower-beds and stuff. I just asked him if we could get married in his backyard and it saved a lot of money as we didn't have to hire a hotel or a church. Sometimes people drive from the church to the hotel to have a party and I just said, 'Let's do everything in one location.' So we did that there and we had the party there. We had the catering there and it was great. My Dad paid for the booze, my Mum paid for the catering. I should write a book on how to do a budget wedding! When people say they spent 20 or 30 grand on a wedding, well I got my tux for $75 downtown. I got the whole tux, I still have it; 75 bucks in the garment district downtown LA. My wife got her dress for a hundred bucks. The wedding ring I think was about 900 bucks; just a simple diamond that we got downtown in the jewellery district. So we probably paid two grand ourselves. I had my friend DJ it; I picked out all the music. And it was awesome, it was great! We had a Christian minister come and do the wedding. I had all my rock friends there. As soon as we were married we had the Billy Idol song 'White Wedding' playing. We just had a good time and it was great. Then we went to Korea and did a traditional Korean wedding where we dressed in Korean outfits and stuff. That was really cool. After that we went inside and they had a reverend, like a Korean Christian reverend, do it in the Korean way and I had to memorise my lines in Korean, so it was pretty interesting.

DANKO JONES: A small one.

EVAN SEINFELD: My wife and I get married all the time. We've been married about seven or eight times. It can really mean a lot when you have all your friends there and all your relatives are there, but it can also mean a lot when it's just two of you in a spiritual ceremony. My wife and I get married at least once a year to remind ourselves of why we're together and to confirm that we want to be together. Life changes.

JAMES KOTTAK: Short and sweet. No big words and just a few people. Or in Tommy Lee's living room.

JESSE HUGHES: The perfect marriage ceremony would be where I marry Carmen Electra… No, I'm just kidding. For me it's like a simple Baptist outdoor ceremony, old-fashioned preacher style.

ROB PATTERSON: On the beach in Maui at sunset.

TOBY RAND: For me, the beach – something outdoors, definitely. I'd probably wear suit pants, no shoes and a vest.

Should your bandmates be expected to be in your wedding party?

ACEY SLADE: Mine were, but I think it depends on the situation. If you're going for the small thing, if they're not invited they shouldn't take it personally. I'm more of a fan of a small intimate wedding, but as far as bandmates go, if they're your best mates then why not?

ALLISON ROBERTSON: Well I was married and I think that they were. I actually had my sister and another friend, part of the old group, and it probably would have been just two people if I didn't have my band. So yeah! Unless they've done something terribly shitty to you, they should be in your wedding party. The more the merrier. Besides, when you appoint people to your wedding party, they basically just have to do a bunch of crap for you. They're like servants. They organise everything, so it's kind of funny to appoint them.

BLASKO: No.

MOST BANDS DON'T GET ALONG WITH EACH OTHER.

CHIP Z'NUFF: I would think the bandmates would be in the wedding party, absolutely. However, there are a lot of bands I know that might not be best friends with each other but they make great music together and have a good chemistry. If I was going to get married again (I'm not getting married again right now OK. I have a girlfriend though) I would have Steven [Adler] as my best man and I'd have the guys in the band there for sure. I'm not going to do that though because Adler would kill me.

COURTNEY TAYLOR-TAYLOR: Depends how long your band has been together.

DANKO JONES: Yeah... well, it depends if you get along with them. Most bands don't get along with each other. So the ones that you do get along with, yeah. Unless you want to mend fences, then invite them all, as long as they don't get completely sloshed and your in-laws start thinking you're a monster.

DOUG ROBB: They would have been but I have a big family and I decided to have my wedding party be just my close, close family. I didn't want to start bringing in friends and stuff, because if you make it too big people start to get offended or something like that if they get left out.

JAMES KOTTAK: No way!

JESSE HUGHES: No, but they should expect to attend.

JIMMY ASHHURST: I guess it depends on what band you're in. If you're in Wham! I would expect no, but I would; I certainly would. I have that relationship with my guys.

NICKE BORG: I would expect them to be, but they would probably have some other stuff to do. Ha! No, of course. I would probably have Dregen as my best man, and Peder and Johan would be there, like totally proud of me.

ROB PATTERSON: Of course! I'd be pissed if they didn't show up! Especially if it's in Hawaii!

TOBY RAND: Bloody oath, they're my best friends! Actually, hold on – you said *in* the wedding party – no. Ha! I've got brothers for that. If I'm rich enough, I'll have a massive wedding party, so maybe then.

VAZQUEZ: No. I would never have a wedding where there'd be like a wedding party, but they'd be invited. They'd probably show up with no gifts.

MASTURBATION
(AUTOEROTICISM)

"DON'T COME INSIDE OF THEM;
IT'S DISRESPECTFUL - SO
PUT IT IN THEIR MOUTH"

What have you discovered about yourself through masturbation?

ACEY SLADE: That I do it entirely too much.

ADDE: That I've got a dirty mind. That I get off on… When you play in a band, you talk with your band members and they're like, 'I get off on this and that' and I see myself as that's not what I'm getting off on and they're like, 'What kind of fantasies do you have?' Well, it's my fantasies.

ANDREW W.K.: Pretty much everything I experienced sexually started with myself. I went through many different ways of feeling about it because before I'd ever been with another girl I had no other experience and really only had myself to base what felt good on. So it was interesting to learn what I like through what I'd already done with myself. And I really learned over the years what felt good to me through myself and it certainly always feels different to have sex by yourself versus sex with a woman, but at the end of the day I think they're both equal. The only time I felt really bad about pleasuring myself was when the girl I was with took offence to it; everything had to be saved for her. At the time, I really believed that I was doing something less than honourable; that I was somehow being unfaithful. Now I understand (whether you use pornography or not) it's a completely discreet, autonomous type of sexuality that is extremely valuable and important and healthy. I think it's always a good idea to maintain that sexual relationship that you have with yourself and have a partner that understands that it has nothing really to do with them. For better or worse, that's for them to understand and interpret how they're going to, but to think that you can't have a personal sexual relationship any more because you are committed in a relationship with someone else is confusing the whole idea. It's not sex with another person, it's sex with yourself and I don't think it should ever be a threat to a relationship.

BRENT MUSCAT: I guess I first discovered my sexuality through masturbation, because before I ever had sex with a girl, masturbating was the first time I ejaculated, so I guess I kind of discovered how everything works. You get hard and you come for the first time. That was through masturbating.

CHIP Z'NUFF: That you'd better be by yourself because you certainly don't want to get caught in a promiscuous position by yourself. It's very healthy for you to get a couple of bullets out of the chamber once in a while. It's very good for you because I do find that when I'm on the road and I rub one out, the chance of me going out and being promiscuous decreases immensely. I'm not even thinking about that. But you go a week or two without anything and sometimes you're at these shows and you see these good-looking chicks and they're smothering you with the admiration and it's really hard to say no. So I recommend it. I think it's healthy for everybody to rub a little banana juice out once or twice a week.

COURTNEY TAYLOR-TAYLOR: Not much I don't think.

DANKO JONES: My hand is my best friend and my life partner.

DOUG ROBB: That I used to masturbate a lot more. Even masturbation gets old. When I was younger, I couldn't wait to have some alone time; now it's like it doesn't really matter as much. I've discovered that I've never been caught masturbating and I think I might be the only one out of all my friends. It seems like in everybody's life, at some point, they get caught – like their Dad walks in or something. So I guess I've noticed through masturbation that I have good planning skills.

EVAN SEINFELD: That too much is never enough.

HANDSOME DICK MANITOBA: I've discovered that I love it, but I don't know what I've ever discovered about myself. I've never really thought about it but it's always been a constant in my life, whether I'm 'getting it' or not, so to speak. It almost doesn't matter. It's almost like sex with another person and masturbation are two separate categories.

JESSE HUGHES: Sex is rad is what I discovered through masturbation.

JIMMY ASHHURST: That I'm fucking hot!

LEMMY: The first thing I discovered was I can have orgasms. Everything else is just details, isn't it?

NICKE BORG: Nothing, I guess. It's just something you do; sometimes I overdo it if I'm frustrated.

ROB PATTERSON: That I'm impatient. Ha!

TOBY RAND: That I like visuals and I like to remember specific women that I've been with and moments in time to get me aroused. And also, it's always good to hold off and not just fucking knock one out really quickly. It's a lot more fun to test yourself to see how far you can go because it always works in the bedroom as well.

VAZQUEZ: I feel that for me, porn has been a really positive thing in my life because I would have never really understood all the things that I truly love about women. I would have never got to understand all that until I got to experience that through porn.

How many times in a day would be considered too many?

ACEY SLADE: I'd say twice. I don't do that any more, but at certain points in my life…

ADDE: Twice actually. I can't masturbate more than one time a day.

ALLISON ROBERTSON: I think that more than once a day is maybe too many.

ANDREW W.K.: I don't know that there's any specific number of too many; it's only when doing it begins to interfere with your ability to do other things that you want to do. Like any addiction, if it gets compulsive to an extent where you're unable to do what you otherwise would in life, then that's probably too many times.

BLASKO: There isn't too many. I suppose it's too many whenever you start bleeding, then you've crossed the line.

BRENT MUSCAT: I remember a friend of mine telling me that he does it a crazy amount of times and I was like, 'How could you do it that many times?' I think he said something like ten times. I remember him telling me he was sore and stuff, so I think if you're making yourself sore, I think that might be too many. I think it might be time to take a break. I think the most I ever did it in a day was probably three times. I think I made myself sore at that time, so I think that would be a point where it's too much and time to give it a break.

CHIP Z'NUFF: Well, I don't want to mention any band names but I know a lot of guys who do it two or three times a day. I recommend if you don't have that big of a sex drive, once a day should be good for you.

COURTNEY TAYLOR-TAYLOR: I would say over four of five you're probably going to wear a hole in it. It should only be if it's a particularly happening part of your life, like a few days in a row where something is happening with you. You're just happening, you're the man, you're on fire or you're so fucking tragically depressed. A little short spell, like a week at the most, of four or five times a day, but I think after that one arm's going to start getting huge! And you're just going to rub a hole in it.

DANKO JONES: More than twice is crazy, or more than three times I guess. That's when you've got to get out of the house dude. Fuck.

DOUG ROBB: It depends on your age: if you're 17 years old and you tell me you masturbate twice a day every day – maybe I've forgotten what it's like to be 17 – I'd be like, 'Dude, that's kind of a lot.' Once a day, if you're young and virile, seems like it should be enough. I think if you're my age of 34 and you're still going more than once a day, you need to get out or find some hobbies or something.

EVAN SEINFELD: Me personally, if I'm separated from my wife for the day, it's not unusual for me to masturbate four or five times on an average day. You know, because my wife and I have sex five or six times a day. I think it's definitely healthy for a man to release himself at least once or twice a day. I think women who masturbate are way more in touch with their orgasm and enjoy sex more. So ladies, don't be shy, just do it.

HANDSOME DICK MANITOBA: It depends how old you are.

JAMES KOTTAK: I'd say 12.

JESSE HUGHES: Whatever amount gets you caught is too many.

JIMMY ASHHURST: Oh God, there's some days when you wonder what the neighbours would think. I don't think there's too many, man; whatever turns you on. That's what we're here for.

LEMMY: Two hundred is too many. I always try and stop at 145, but it depends on your age I think. When you're younger, you do it a lot more but as you get older you do it less, or you want to do it less somehow.

NICKE BORG: Six hours in a row.

ROB PATTERSON: Eight.

TOBY RAND: I don't think there is such a thing as too many. If you can do it many times a day why wouldn't you fucking do it? I think it's probably a reason why rock stars knock back groupies because they've been wanking a lot on the tour bus.

VAZQUEZ: I think that it depends on the individual. For me, I'll rub one out like once a day if I know I'm not getting laid.

Is it a turn-on to watch someone masturbate?

ACEY SLADE: Watching a girl masturbate? For sure, that is really a turn-on.

ADDE: Yeah, absolutely!

ALLISON ROBERTSON: For me it's not. For me it's definitely not. I don't know why. Maybe I'm weird, but it isn't.

BLASKO: Another girl – yes.

DANKO JONES: Not a dude, not for me! But yeah, it is I guess. It depends on your state of arousal. It could be like, 'This is boring the shit out of me.'

EVAN SEINFELD: A woman, yeah.

GINGER: Hell yeah! It's also the perfect way to find out exactly how they like it.

IF YOU ARE MASTURBATING IN A ROOM WITH SOMEONE ELSE, THAT'S NOT QUITE TRUE MASTURBATION; YOU'RE SHARING IT WITH SOMEONE, SO IT BREAKS THAT BOND OF SELF.

HANDSOME DICK MANITOBA: Yeah, I love that kind of sexual play with my girl. Sometimes we'll play with ourselves separately. To me though, the masturbatory act is when you're alone in a room. If you are masturbating in a room with someone else, that's not quite true masturbation; you're sharing it with someone, so it breaks that bond of self. But it's something that I'll always do and I've always done and I'll always enjoy. It almost has nothing to do with getting it or not getting it, whether I'm happy or not. It's a nice comfort thing; it's always there for you.

JAMES KOTTAK: No.

JESSE HUGHES: So long as it's not a dude, it's a total turn-on for me.

JIMMY ASHHURST: A female, yeah. Very much so.

LEMMY: No. Can you see every question you've asked me is personal; do all the chicks really like that? It all depends on your mother and father, unless you're Sigmund Freud.

NICKE BORG: Yeah, for sure – absolutely!

ROB PATTERSON: Of course! My girl though; not some dude!

TOBY RAND: Yeah, I love watching a girl masturbate.

VAZQUEZ: Kind of… like, as soon as I start seeing it I'm like, 'OK, I'm ready to get going.' It's not like I want to sit there and watch her play with herself, it's like, 'OK, now I want to fuck you.'

What's best to do with the semen after masturbating?

ACEY SLADE: On a bus you use a sock, for sure. Have you ever heard of sock races? If you're in your band and nobody got laid that night, everybody jumps in their bunk and jacks off. Then whoever throws their sock into the aisle first is the loser. Now, I've never had this actual experience before, but I've heard of it. I personally don't want to know when another guy is jacking off.

ADDE: Give it to her on the breasts, or in the mouth. Yeah!

ANDREW W.K.: I would say dispose of it somehow. I wouldn't leave it sitting around, or hanging around. I have had friends who really got off on semen left on their clothes and going about their day. Again, I thought that was really aggressive. It reminded me of sex in public or sex where other people can hear you. It's an aggressive violation of other people's desire to be involved with you sexually; like flashing somebody.

BLASKO: Clean it up and get rid of it right away.

BRENT MUSCAT: Well you could do anything with it really. You could shoot it somewhere, put it in a tissue, grab a shirt that you need to wash. I don't know what's best to do with it. I guess just try not to get it on something that someone could see later. Too much on your bed sheets could be embarrassing if you have a girlfriend or friend over. So I guess just a tissue or a warm wash cloth is good.

CHIP Z'NUFF: If you're by yourself, make sure you've got a towel or a baby sock or something so you don't make a big mess. Then discard it instantly, in the washing machine immediately, or if you're in a hotel in the garbage can. If you're with a woman, you know where to put it. Just discard it. Don't come inside of them; it's disrespectful – so put it in their mouth. If you feel like you're going to finish, just tell her and do it that way. I think that's still enjoyable and there's no mess.

COURTNEY TAYLOR-TAYLOR: Toilet. I'm going to go with a towel or

whatever. You don't want that to go down the drain; it's going to create plumbing hazards. It's probably going to cost you $140 to collect the hairballs that have collected around your jizz, so don't let that go down the drain. It goes in the toilet, hopefully clinging together with some kind of paper or whatever, or just do it in the towel.

DANKO JONES: Clean it up. Get up, go to the washroom and clean yourself

off. That's what I always do.

DOUG ROBB: Don't use it as hair gel! Throw it away if it's in a paper towel or

a tissue or whatever. Dirty clothes are always good to clean it up with because you're washing the clothes anyway.

JAMES KOTTAK: Clean it up!

JESSE HUGHES: It's best to clean it up and get rid of it completely.

JIMMY ASHHURST: A quick and graceful disposal. A good toilet flushing is

probably the best.

LEMMY: Oh, chuck it away man. It's no good keeping it.

NICKE BORG: If you don't want to get caught by doing it in your kitchen, you

just fucking try to have something to contain it in and throw it away. If you're with someone else, maybe you let it be on that person if she wants to. It depends on how many times you did it before, so maybe it doesn't come out that much.

ROB PATTERSON: Swallow it.

TOBY RAND: For me, it's either to already have an old T-shirt ready to go

or just wipe it into your body like it's moisturiser. But one of my friends actually devours it – no names mentioned. Not that I've seen him do it, but yeah, it's fucking weird.

VAZQUEZ: I jerk off on the toilet so I just fire it right into the toilet and I'm

done. It's efficient, it's clean, everybody's happy.

How can the best orgasm be achieved by masturbating?

ACEY SLADE: With porn, or with another partner there.

BLASKO: The longer you can hold out, the better.

JIMMY ASHHURST: Foreplay: If you can tease yourself into having some patience, then usually the end result is more voluminous.

ROB PATTERSON: If you don't know this, something is wrong.

TOBY RAND: Grab your balls really tight and when you're about to blow don't actually stroke it, just hold the base of your cock and your balls just before you blow and then afterwards keep on pulling yourself.

VAZQUEZ: For me, as long as I've got some porn, I'm fine. I just switched to videos. I used to be into magazines for some reason and then I started getting into videos and I'm more into that now. I don't know why I was into magazines for so long. People were like, 'Why do you fucking buy those?' and I'm like, 'I don't know man, I just like it.'

MONEY FOR SEX

"USUALLY THEY'RE NOT EVEN HALF AS HORNY AS THE GIRL NEXT DOOR, BUT THERE IS SOMETHING KIND OF ROMANTIC ABOUT ROCK'N'ROLL AND STRIP CLUBS"

How would you select a prostitute at a brothel?

ACEY SLADE: Just go for the hottest one – easy.

BLASKO: I've never been to one so I don't know. But for my money, she'd have to be the hottest.

BRENT MUSCAT: Pick the least attractive one because she's probably going to be the one most willing to please you and in some ways I think she's probably going to be the cleanest one. Chances are the best looking one has probably had too much sex that day and is not going to be into it.

CHANCES ARE THE BEST LOOKING ONE HAS PROBABLY HAD TOO MUCH SEX THAT DAY AND IS NOT GOING TO BE INTO IT.

CHIP Z'NUFF: I've been to brothels before. All the girls come up to you and they talk to you at the bar while you're ordering a drink and you just can tell by the way they carry themselves, the tone of their voice, the words they use, what they have to say to you, how they say it – that's everything. It's pretty easy to pick them. Don't just go by the looks. Make sure you have a real conversation. It's very important and that'll ease any doubts you have about that person. I recommend conversation first for a few minutes and then, of course, look at her. Make sure she trips your trigger face-wise and everything else and then you'll know. Remember when you're in those brothels you've got a choice. There's usually between 10 to 30 girls there. You've got plenty of time. Be patient – patience is a virtue. If you're there looking for that, you'll eventually find something that you can work with and make it work with you.

COURTNEY TAYLOR-TAYLOR: I've never paid for sex, but from what I've seen with friends is you just walk around until one of them gives you that electric impulse in your lower abdomen that just makes you go, 'Holy shit! Wow, I need to come now.' Don't expect it to be great. It's clinical and they're going to go for more money. They're just going to be trying to grab your wallet. Some will almost get you there and then go for your wallet trying to get more like, 'C'mon, c'mon, another, another.' So you've got to be a hair trigger guy anyway since you're paying for it. It's a job.

DANKO JONES: She's got to be hot I guess, really hot. I don't think I'd do it. Personally, I would not do that, but if I was to do it I would make sure she was a fine, physical specimen.

DOUG ROBB: That's another thing I've never experienced, but if I had to I would probably just go for the one I thought was most physically attractive. I mean, isn't that what you do?

HANDSOME DICK MANITOBA: I've been to prostitutes three times in my life: one time was when The Dictators were in Amsterdam in '78 I think, or '77. We walked around and there were some of them that were drop-dead gorgeous but they wanted a ridiculous amount of money. Then there were some that were girls-next-door that were cute enough. What we did was we all found one and separated and said, 'Let's meet in an hour' and that was it. I picked one and went. Next time was when I was driving a cab in New York City and I picked up a callgirl in Central Park West and she kept talking about it saying, 'C'mon, C'mon!' She talked me into doing something in the cab. And the third time was my 27th birthday and that was it. I just happened to stumble into these situations; it wasn't like, 'I'm going to go pick one out.'

JAMES KOTTAK: Whoever had the most recent shower.

JESSE HUGHES: I've never been with a prostitute in my life.

JIMMY ASHHURST: We have the internet for that nowadays. There was a time in Thailand where they all were numbered, which I thought was quite handy. It made it easier. Like, 'I'll have a number seven with a side of number 13.'

LEMMY: I don't know; I've never been to one. I'd just like to say, I don't understand how it can be illegal to sell something that's perfectly legal to give away. It's a stupid law, which takes up a lot of cop hours and puts a lot of people in jail for no reason. If someone wants to get laid, they're going to get laid, whether you put the chick in jail first time you catch them or not.

NICKE BORG: Well they all say they want to marry you and that they love you, so depending on how many drinks you've had, it's up to you to believe it or not. But I've actually been in situations where they say, 'You're so fucking awesome. I love you. My name is Angel Rose.' And I'm like, 'No you're not.' 'No, seriously, my name is Lydia Garcena.' 'No it's not.' 'Well it is; here's my cell phone number.' And I'm like, 'No, it's not' and it was. So, you never know. But dude, you have to be so fucked up to go and find a prostitute at a fucking whorehouse or whatever and want to pay to have sex. I guess there's something kind of kinky about it, but I would never recommend it – no.

ROB PATTERSON: Never done it.

TOBY RAND: I've never been to a brothel. Well, I've been to one but never had a prostitute… but if I was to, I would select the hottest looking one. It's not like I'm going to be hanging out with her.

Do strippers make good sexual partners?

ACEY SLADE: Yeah they do; they make good sexual partners but probably not long-term.

ADDE: Yeah, absolutely!

ALLISON ROBERTSON: Yeah I think they can. I think it completely depends on someone's skill level. It has nothing to do with what they do as a job, or how sexy or unsexy their job is. I think it totally depends on how you're attracted to them or whatever.

BLASKO: I've known them to be and I've known them not to be. I think there's a mythology involved with the presentation in the sense that you look and go, 'Oh, that's going to be hot in the sack' and sometimes it's not. Sometimes you want to sue for false advertising.

BRENT MUSCAT: Not necessarily. I know a lot of strippers are jaded. From my understanding, strippers who have been at it a long time see a certain type of guy in the club who are looking at their body and just looking for sex. But I don't think all the guys are like that. Sometimes these girls get a preconceived idea of how guys are, so with some of them the last thing they want to do is have sex. Not all of them are like that though. I've had fun with some and had sex with some who have been a lot of fun, but from my experience there's a lot of them who have got some guy issues. So I wouldn't say they do it better; it really just depends on the girl.

CHIP Z'NUFF: No. They're great dancers and I love the art form. I appreciate them and I love them. They're great all around the country; they're really nice. It's a tough job to be a stripper and I love strippers. But the ones I've been with have been very selfish and they're consumed with themselves and time is money.

COURTNEY TAYLOR-TAYLOR: Not that I've experienced but I don't know, that's just me. I've had very limited sexual experiences with strippers that I know of. I'm sure that any member of Mötley Crüe would just go, 'You're fucking crazy! What the fuck did he just say? Hey dude, you're never going to believe what this idiot just fucking said!'

DANKO JONES: I suppose. I don't go out with strippers, but I know many guys who have and do and what I've been told is their work environment has a sexual atmosphere that's so heightened, more than any other work environment. That's where they are all day, it's got to translate in the bedroom. From what I've been told, it does. What I've heard about it is there are a lot more fetishes that crop up that they want, just because I think that occupation attracts a certain personality. I've heard of some weird shit and it makes sense because of their occupation.

DOUG ROBB: I don't know; I've never had a sexual partner who was a stripper… that I know of.

GINGER: In my personal experience, strippers use sex as a workout or sport. Nothing lacks spontaneity more than someone with their moves already worked out.

HANDSOME DICK MANITOBA: I hate to sound intellectual in a book that's fun, but there's like 50 million strippers in the world and I don't think you can make a statement that because they do that they're good or they're bad; it's too simplistic. I think there are probably women who hate men because they do that. I think there are women who probably do it as part of their life and if they find the right guy they can be great partners, and there's probably women who are terrible partners because of it. I think it's the same gamut as any other business; I think some people are ruined by it and some people aren't.

JAMES KOTTAK: I wouldn't know, but all they want is your money so don't bother.

JESSE HUGHES: Not in my opinion, but of course anyone can make a good sexual partner. I'm personally not into it.

JIMMY ASHHURST: There was a time in Hollywood when me and my buddies knew one in at least every part of town, so we'd end up at whichever bar and it'd be the one that was from the closest bar that would end up entertaining us all for the evening. As you grow older and hopefully become more successful, I think the whole stripper thing loses its intrigue. I got tired of paying for the boyfriend's Playstation games who was sitting at home waiting for her to get back with the cash. So once you've been that guy, you tend to be a bit wary of it later on.

LEMMY: Usually no because they're usually going out with another chick in the troupe or they… In a strip club, you don't meet the best, classy guys usually – they're more like gross, animal, pigs you know? So that doesn't endear the male sex to the chicks really. Working as a stripper doesn't do anything for the promotion of the male as a suitable sexual partner. It's a shame.

NICKE BORG: Anyone who wants to take their clothes off in front of a lot of strange men (or strange girls, whatever) to get some dollars tucked into their panties or between their cheeks has a little of something wrong in their head in a way, I guess. Usually they're not even half as horny as the girl next door, but there is something kind of romantic about rock'n'roll and strip clubs. I usually go to strip clubs, and I really like to go to strip clubs. Sometimes I just go there for the vibe, the drinks, the whole tacky Seventies/Eighties vibe that you usually don't find these days… and sometimes they play good rock'n'roll music as well. Sometimes I like to hang out with strippers because when it comes down to it, they're not even interested in having sex, which sometimes is relieving.

TOBY RAND: Yeah they do. I've dated strippers before. The good thing about them is that they have a lot of fun – their job is fun. They're pretty much like rock stars; they go on stage and people watch them, so they don't have any inhibitions. They love exhibitionism and don't seem to have any qualms getting their gear off and having fucking fun.

Is it better to pay for sex on the road, or masturbate?

ACEY SLADE: I think if you're paying for sex, you're cheating. If that's what you're trying to get around, masturbating or paying for it; if you're paying for it, you're cheating. It's not cheating unless you're paying for it, so if you're trying to stay faithful, then obviously masturbating. But if you're on the road and you're not trying to be faithful, I don't see any reason why you would have to pay for it anyway.

ADDE: If you meet a girl at the bar and you buy her drinks all night, just keep her interested. That's pretty much like a hidden prostitution to me, so I don't care too much for that.

BLASKO: If you're married, certainly masturbation is the way to go.

DANKO JONES: It's cheaper, it's easier, it's cleaner, it's just less drama and everything to masturbate. It's just way easier and you save your per diems.

ROB PATTERSON: Definitely masturbate!

TOBY RAND: I haven't paid for sex yet, which means I'm pretty lucky, so I'll just have a groupie instead.

Any tips for getting best value for money?

EVAN SEINFELD: We're up against a similar animal as Napster, Limewire and all those music peer-to-peer sites in the adult business. It's really tough on the business but I will say this: when all porn is free, no one will be able to make quality porn any more. We're all going to have to watch fat, ugly people have sex. So if you're a fan of Tera Patrick, or whatever you're a fan of, join their websites, support them, and help them be able to give you the quality entertainment you'd like to have.

WHEN ALL PORN IS FREE, NO ONE WILL BE ABLE TO MAKE QUALITY PORN ANY MORE. WE'RE ALL GOING TO HAVE TO WATCH FAT, UGLY PEOPLE HAVE SEX.

ROB PATTERSON: Yeah, don't spend it!

How can one choose a good phone sex service?

BLASKO: Do those even exist any more? I have no clue.

DANKO JONES: Those are really expensive. I find phone sex is great with someone who you know. It's just way better.

ROB PATTERSON: I have no idea. The phone book? The LA Weekly massage section?

TOBY RAND: The only experience I've had is just prank calls with my mates on the road, totally just for fun – shits and giggles. So just choose whatever.

What city in the world has the best sex workers?

ACEY SLADE: Probably Cologne in Germany. The Reeperbahn in Cologne is really cool. I like it better than Amsterdam because the Amsterdam one is just like everywhere man, whereas in Cologne there's like one strip where the girls are in the windows and it's pretty cool.

ALLISON ROBERTSON: I'd probably have to say Japan and maybe Sweden and Germany, just because it's such a big deal in those places and people get really specific that you'd probably have to be really skilled. And I'd even throw LA into there, on the private tips – the private for hire.

BLASKO: I would have to assume Amsterdam. I've never even been to Amsterdam, but I would have to assume there just because it's like that's where it all is. It's got a lot to live up to that's for sure.

BRENT MUSCAT: There were a few places in Europe that I went to that had red light districts and some of the girls seemed pretty good-looking there. I don't know. I've never really been attracted to girls who I have to pay for. Maybe I was spoiled because I was in the band and never really had to pay for it, or I've always had a girlfriend anyway.

CHIP Z'NUFF: I love Scores in New York – Scores East and West. Last time we did a major radio show over there the DJ set us up and that was a really good place. I love it over there. People are really friendly and they really take care of you these girls. You can drink your ass off and there are pretty much no rules and regulations. If you trip the girls' trigger, they'll go back to your place with you and hang out and kick it.

COURTNEY TAYLOR-TAYLOR: Amsterdam, it really does. It really has all kinds. You want smart girls that talk to you? I think you can pretty much find it. I talked to some lady. She was bored, I was bored. She was in her window; I was standing there in front of the little pub next door waiting for somebody. God, she was cool. Just really hot. She was probably late thirties or something and my God, crazy. If you can achieve it, I imagine the best way to choose a chick in a brothel is if you can honestly, with no hint of irony, turn to your buddy and go, 'I would date her.' That would be the best of all. That's the tier one echelon. From what I understand though, it rarely happens.

DANKO JONES: I guess it would be Amsterdam because it's legal and people go there just to do that. Having walked through the red lights, there are a lot of hot girls out there in the red lights. Some of them are so hot you just kind of go, 'What the fuck are you doing here?' But now I know you should avoid them. I didn't really think about that.

DOUG ROBB: It's probably a cliché to say Amsterdam but it's definitely the first place I've walked around and been really exposed to public sex for sale. I've been there when a couple of my crew guys indulged and I asked them about it and even they thought it's a little strange. Maybe it's because in the States in the most part it's completely illegal, so it's hard to wrap their heads around it. We did go to this district in Bangkok and we went into this club or something like that and we sat around what looked like a bar. About 20 girls were just pseudo-dancing, just stepping back and forth in bikinis. They had numbers on their bikinis and I saw people going like, 'Yeah, I'll take number 37!' and just walk off. That's pretty serious. So I'd say Amsterdam or Bangkok.

JAMES KOTTAK: I'm sure Amsterdam.

JESSE HUGHES: I have not had sex with a prostitute but I've put one to work easily a couple of times. Let me explain this to you: it was at the very old Marriott hotel in Warsaw, Poland and I walked into the bar and I shit you not, there was probably a seven to one ratio of women to men. The hottest Euro-porn worthy, 19 to 22-year-old girls playing the bar and it was like $30 a girl (USD-equivalent) for whatever you wanted. I took three of them up to a friend's room and we made them slip tricks like ponies, you know what I'm saying?

JIMMY ASHHURST: Toronto. And of course the more well-known one: Amsterdam. Window shopping is kind of an amazing concept. We haven't quite become that civilised in my country yet, unfortunately.

LEMMY: I don't know. I've never had one, you see? Not on duty anyway.

NICKE BORG: Los Angeles… and Austin, Texas.

ROB PATTERSON: I'm guessing Amsterdam from what I've been told.

TOBY RAND: Going from other people's experience, it has to be Amsterdam. Personally, I have seen Thailand and yeah… awesome.

VAZQUEZ: I've never really done that, so if I had to guess… isn't like Amsterdam the big deal with that? That's what I hear anyway. In the US there's not really a lot of brothels per se, they have more escort services and shit like that.

ONE-NIGHT STANDS

"WITH A BEANIE, SOME SPECTACLES AND A MASSIVE COAT I WAS ABLE TO ESCAPE WITH ALL MY PARTS INTACT"

How should you let them know you're only looking for a one-night stand?

ACEY SLADE: I think if a girl's hooking up with a guy in a band and it's the first night, she should pretty much take it for granted that it's going to be a one-night stand. I think it's kind of an unspoken thing, but then again that comes back to the younger versus older thing; a more mature girl's going to know that. And there's nothing wrong with a girl wanting to bang a hot guy she saw on stage every once in a while.

ADDE: It's kind of obvious: if you're at the bar that's pretty much a one-night stand.

ALLISON ROBERTSON: I think just say it right away so you don't have to deal with them crying later, you know what I mean? Kind of tell them, 'Hey, this is just for tonight.'

ANDREW W.K.: People have often been really surprised that I haven't ever really taken advantage of my profession as it traditionally… It's really fascinated me with the people who have, to the point of debauchery. It's really interesting, like, 'What drives someone to that? What holds someone else back from that?' To be quite honest, I really think the only difference is – I would love to have had, and in many ways to still have and maybe I will, even though I'm married anything's possible; my wife is very open-minded – the idea of having lots and lots of one-night stands basically is a theory that appeals to me very much, much like pornography; that's what I get out of pornography. The emotional, social and ethical side of one-night stands is where I have trouble, meaning I don't know how that would feel to me or that person over the long run and thinking of what you end up going through after that rush of the physical moment.

BLASKO: I don't think I've ever been clear on that issue. Sometimes it comes to bite you in the ass – actually more times than not. Sometimes it's an understood thing and it's all good, no one's feeling guilty about it. Prior to getting married, I never knew and I still don't know that there's a good way to do that.

BRENT MUSCAT: I don't think you necessarily have to let them know that. From my point of view, if I was touring and I was in a city and I'm leaving the next day, it's kind of common knowledge or just assumed. It's like, 'Well you know I'm leaving tomorrow right?' There were times where if I really liked the girl I'd keep her number and every time I'd go to that city I'd call her up. I don't think it's necessarily something you have to discuss. I don't think it would be a very good ice-breaker if you said, 'Hey baby, I only want to have sex with you the once.' That could ruin your whole plans.

CHIP Z'NUFF: I don't think you let them know. I think you just leave it alone. If you're with somebody and it's going to happen and you just met each other, just give it everything you've got. The more questions you ask, the deeper you're going to find yourself in. Pretty much, if you meet that person and you both like each other, do your thing and leave it alone. Don't ask, don't tell – I like that.

COURTNEY TAYLOR-TAYLOR: The best possible way is just the nature of your job description: I am a singer in a rock band. We tour the world, a lot. That's pretty much the best way for me. Basically, I've never really hooked up with anyone that I wasn't kind of hoping was going to be my girlfriend. The only times that it ever then became an issue was due to geography. Then you just kind of know that it might be a yearly thing or twice-a-year thing if you like them and they come through. I really doubt if people generally go and… I don't know what other people do, never mind. I never had to let anyone know that, 'You know, last night was just last night. I don't actually like you and I don't ever want to do that again.' I've never had that situation at all.

DANKO JONES: Yeah that's interesting. It depends where this one-night stand happens. If it happens at a bar and it's just you and someone that you met, I guess it's kind of understood that there's a certain percentage that this is just going to be a one-night stand between the two of you. If it happens at a show and it's a one-night stand, the person (not the one in the band but the other one) might misconstrue and she might show up the next night.

DOUG ROBB: Do you have to? Can't you just leave? Wouldn't that be easiest, to just leave?

GINGER: Always tell them beforehand. It's worth risking losing a shag beforehand than having to deal with the uncomfortable proposition of getting rid of someone afterwards.

HANDSOME DICK MANITOBA: It depends how you go into the situation, where you met, what you're looking for. Read the signs. You've got instincts for a reason. You've got eyes and ears for a reason. You've got a brain for a reason. Read the signs. There's been times where it's been the other way around. Like when I was looking to fool around with this girl and she took me to her father's box at the Giants football game and I put my hand on her knee and she's like, 'Oh, I don't want to lead you the wrong way.' And I'm going like, 'I'm 30-something years old, you took me on a date, I'm a man, you're a woman.' It's good to just say that shit, 'I'm looking for this, you're looking for this, we're looking for two different things.' No one's right or wrong. It's like, everybody's in a different place. You can have the right person in your life, but if it's the wrong time, it's the wrong person. It's all about a certain rightness. I think you've just got to let people know where you're at. You don't have to make a speech. Read the signs, everybody should just read the damn signs.

JAMES KOTTAK: As soon as the deed is done, split!

JESSE HUGHES: It depends: if lying to them is required then you do so and you let them know by the fact that you haven't called in six weeks and you don't return any text messages. Nine times out of 10 it's very difficult for a dude to just be straight-up about that. They've always got to come in with an angle because unfortunately most men look at sex as getting something from a girl as opposed to doing it with. You get laid, you get some action. But when you look at it like that, normally it requires a woman to say, 'Look dude, I don't give a fuck if you don't call me.'

JIMMY ASHHURST: I'm terrible at that man, I really am. The more times that you can repeat that you're leaving in the morning would be a good start. Maybe leaving a plane ticket on the nightstand or something.

JOEL O'KEEFFE: Say something like, 'The bus leaves in four hours babe, so it's now or never.' Even if the bus doesn't, it guarantees you an escape option.

LEMMY: The ones who are willing to do it, that's all they usually want anyway. It's just a bit of an adventure thing really. I like one-night stands; they're great! I even wrote a song about it.

NICKE BORG: I think that depends on how it went. I think you are in just as much big trouble as well if you think you just want to fuck that chick, then get away and catch the bus to the next city with your band. If she turns out to be, 'Jesus fucking Christ man, she's so great!', you thought that you were using her but she could blow your fucking mind by being the greatest fucking chick you've ever met in your life – at least at the time you think that. I think we all expect it to be one night though, especially if you meet someone after 12 o'clock night time, but sometimes you surprise yourself by being fucked by the greatest girl.

ROB PATTERSON: I've only had two in my life, and it was just understood from the beginning.

TOBY RAND: I think for starters, when you're on the road, it's pretty obvious you're going to the next city the next night and you make it quite clear to them that you'll be leaving in the morning. Other than that, it's just a case of telling them, 'You seem like an awesome person so let's have fucking fun for one night and remember it forever.'

VAZQUEZ: You've got to be honest with them right up front; you've got to tell them. The beautiful thing about a one-night stand when you're on tour is like any new relationship, but instead of it happening over the course of say a year or two, it happens in the course of hours! You have that first meeting, you have that little courtship, you have that little bit of foreplay, you have that whole sex and everything else, then you have that tearful goodbye. It's weird man, because you do end up having that mini-relationship.

What's the best way to let them down gently the next morning and escape?

ACEY SLADE: Say, 'I've got bus call.'

ADDE: First of all, I go to their place. I don't want to bring them to my place; I go to their place and then I don't leave my phone number or anything. I just say like, 'Thank you so much, you're wonderful and see you later. Bye.'

DON'T STICK AROUND AND COOK BREAKFAST! JUST GET THE FUCK OUT AS FAST AS YOU CAN.

ALLISON ROBERTSON: I would probably pull the 'I have a boyfriend at home.' It might piss somebody off but then they really know that they don't have a chance. Because if you say anything like, 'Next time…' or lead them on to make them think there will be a next time in general and you don't want that, then in my experience you'll get a stalker situation. So it's almost better to lie and say you're gay and that was just for fun. It seems like that might be better than saying, 'Oh yeah, that was really fun. Next time I'm in town…' Nobody likes feeling like that person's coming back and when they do come back they ignore you; it feels really bad if you're on the other end of that. I don't know. You don't want to waste people's time.

CHIP Z'NUFF: Just be honest and say, 'I'm ready to go to the next city. I had a wonderful time with you last night. God bless you and your family. I hope to see you again soon. Ta-ta.'

DANKO JONES: I'm really bad at that. Just avoid or play stupid. I guess, no matter how much you've been backed up against the wall, at the end of the day, it's just to be very honest with someone no matter how much it hurts. Once you get it out, it's actually a lot easier. This girl, I guess we misunderstood each other, and I was like, 'I was thinking it was this but obviously you were thinking it was this way. I'm really sorry.' Usually they don't accept your apology and probably leave a ton of hateful messages on boards or forums. The times there have been misunderstandings with me, I've just never been able to talk to that person and sort it out because you're gone – you're here one day and then you're gone – you're always travelling. Whether the one-night stand happened at home or on the road or whatever, and this is what really bothers me, you're never able to get that person in a corner and just have them hear you out. Usually it's just too late by the time you see them again. They've been thinking about it for all those weeks, months, or even a year or two and you cannot convince them otherwise. It's just an uphill battle that you might as well forget about. That's one thing that really bugs me about being in a band; you're here one day, gone the next. If someone's talking shit about you or someone misunderstands you, whether it's about sex or anything else, it's so hard to clear your name sometimes. If there's somebody that doesn't like me (I'm not even talking professionally; I'm talking personally) and it's even worse if we actually spent some intimate time together, it really bugs me if they don't like me, because I'm not out to hurt people when it comes to relationships like that. That's just not my style. I'm telling you this because it has happened and I've just never been able to clear my name with a couple of people. It just bugs me.

DOUG ROBB: Don't stick around and cook breakfast! Just get the fuck out as fast as you can. That's the easiest, most blunt symbol of 'I just wanted this once.'

JAMES KOTTAK: Say, 'Oh man, we've got a band meeting that I forgot about.'

JESSE HUGHES: I've let girls down gently in this way: I've said I need to use the bathroom. I go and I turn on the sink and then I push out the screen and sneak out their window with the door locked.

JOEL O'KEEFFE: Well, just say, 'I'm ducking out for a smoke; want anything while I'm gone?' Then run like fuck to the bus and tell the driver to floor it!

LEMMY: You don't have to escape. I mean, you're usually leaving anyway, in my business. I don't know what it's like when you live there all the time. That could get sticky I suppose, in more ways than one.

ROB PATTERSON: Don't wait until the next morning! Go when they fall asleep! Ha.

TOBY RAND: The best escape route is when the tour manager has got a text message from you the night before saying you're with a girl and can you please bang on my door and drag me out, or get her out of the room. And say she has to go because there's an emergency!

How do you avoid further contact?

ACEY SLADE: It's impossible now; it's impossible. Really, you have to be more honest with people now, more than ever because you're going to get nailed if you're cheating on your wife or girlfriend, or something like that. You're going to get nailed one way or another and it's through the internet.

ANDREW W.K.: Well definitely don't give your phone number and if you do, give one that you don't answer. But from the beginning, I think you can just say, 'I'm not going to give you my phone number.' You might not ever talk again. If she freaks out, then hopefully you're not alone with her. The more you can be direct, the better it will be. Sometimes I've had it where girls will just pretend like I didn't say that and have just gone through that whole freak-out anyway.

BLASKO: Don't give them your phone number; don't give them your MySpace, I suppose.

BRENT MUSCAT: Well I guess you have a choice if you want to give them your contact details or not. If you don't want to see them, you don't have to give them your number. You could just say, 'Hey it was nice hanging out with you. Maybe I'll see you next time I'm in town' or something like that.

CHIP Z'NUFF: Well you're busy and you've got a road manager who watches over you and the whole team, so you're in pretty good shape. You might see them again. If you see them again next time, they'll have a good memory from the last time.

COURTNEY TAYLOR-TAYLOR: Here would be the best way to do it: 'Oh, I feel so guilty. Oh my gosh! I have a girlfriend. I'm just feeling so guilty, I thought I should tell you that. It's just that you're so hot, I couldn't help myself. I'd better go now.' That would be a good one I think. 'Please don't tell anyone. I really just couldn't help myself.'

DOUG ROBB: I guess if you're leaving you don't give them any contact info or whatever. If you happened to give them contact info and they try to contact you and you never call them back or anything, I think that's probably the easiest hint.

HANDSOME DICK MANITOBA: I've been there before, but personally, I'm really sensitive to not pushing myself onto someone. Love the ones you're with, love the ones who want you. Don't keep chasing someone. Like, you can chase someone for a little while and if they fall for you, great. But if you keep chasing them, it's almost like idolising someone. I wouldn't move too hard. If I met a new girl, I'd always wait a day or two to call; never be too hungry. There's nothing that turns someone off more than being too hungry or too needy.

JAMES KOTTAK: I don't know any more with all these cell phones and everything else. I don't know.

JESSE HUGHES: Avoid them at all costs and if you see them again, pretend like they're not there.

JIMMY ASHHURST: Saying that you have an imaginary identical twin or doppelganger is good for escape. You can come back to town and say, 'No, no. That wasn't me. That must have been my twin brother.' Especially if anything unsavoury may have occurred. Deny everything.

JOEL O'KEEFFE: Well sometimes further contact is good and better than the first. But if it's not, well then it's time to bust out ninja stealth and evade capture at all costs. The last time I had to employ the art of ninja stealth was on a UK tour. With a beanie, some spectacles and a massive coat, I was able to escape with all my parts intact.

LEMMY: Well listen, if she's that bad, why would you be there in the first place? I've never been with a monster. To avoid contact you just shut everything down.

ROB PATTERSON: Don't give them your contact info!

TOBY RAND: Well for starters she doesn't have your actual phone number. The thing I like to do with a person is to make them feel totally comfortable and not make it weird in the morning. Wake up the next morning and make it fun. You have a little brekky or whatever it is, or you say you've got shit to do and you just be honest with them and say, 'Listen, I'm not looking for anything, just a bit of fun.' I think it's always good to run off and avoid it, but it always comes back to bite you. I reckon dealing with it right then and there and saying you're here for a bit of fun seems to work.

VAZQUEZ: Diplomacy and discretion – if you don't use that then you're going to have a lot of problems.

ORAL SEX

"DON'T MESS AROUND TOO MUCH WITH IT, LIKE LOOK AT IT OR BLOW ON IT OR PLAY WITH IT. IF YOU'RE GOING TO SUCK IT, PUT IT IN YOUR MOUTH AND SUCK IT"

Is there a never-fail mouth technique for blowjobs that takes you over the edge?

ACEY SLADE: Girls underestimate the hand a lot when it comes to a blowjob; there's nothing worse than a girl who's just bobbing up and down with her mouth. The hand has to be used; it has to, especially if they're twisting it.

ADDE: Loads of spit. Yeah, loads of spit!

ALLISON ROBERTSON: No, I don't think so. I think you just have to have really nice lips. I know this seems obvious, but I know a lot of girls I talk to still don't really like it. They lie and say they do, but they don't. So I think that has a lot to do with it. If you just don't like it, you don't like it, but you usually have to eventually. One thing I notice that I think is funny is that a lot of women don't seem to have grasped to just be careful about the teeth. C'mon! You're supposed to have learned that in grade school. I think that's the number one rule.

ANDREW W.K.: Yes, going slowly. It's been a big misunderstanding for a lot of girls that it's not about trying to simulate traditional vaginal intercourse. It's totally something unique and different and a lot of it has to do with the visual side, a lot of it has to do with having this different point of view and just taking one's time, and going slowly I think also could be more comfortable for the girl. That's always worked for me.

BLASKO: It's like, people ask and say, 'I'm not that good at it.' Well the bottom line is this: as long as you're doing it, you're off to a good start and if you just don't involve any teeth in it, then it's all good.

BRENT MUSCAT: If the girl can deep throat then that's always fun. If they can take in as much as they can that's always kind of sexy, at least for me. Maybe that's a fetish, I don't know. For me, if you're going to do it, just do it. Don't mess around too much with it, like look at it or blow on it or play with it. If you're going to suck it, put it in your mouth and suck it. The whole thing of trying to be cute and doing this or doing that is not for me. If you're going to do it, stick it in your mouth and suck on it.

CHIP Z'NUFF: Yeah I like the use of the hand also, like a motorcycle throttle turning the hand at the same time. We call it the Pepper Shaker or the Motorcycle Throttle. For anybody, unless you have a really good mind-set, that puts you over the top, right there. That gets the ball rolling instantly. However, you've got to be careful because you can let one out of the chamber, then you're doomed for a while because it's not like us men are all 18 years old, where we're that resilient that we can get a rig right away again. But the Motorcycle Throttle at the same time is the best technique.

COURTNEY TAYLOR-TAYLOR: No, I don't think so.

DANKO JONES: It's got to be mouth and hand. That works perfectly. No teeth; mouth and hand.

DOUG ROBB: I think just the sloppier the better.

HANDSOME DICK MANITOBA: Nah, no tricks. It's all in the moment. It's all a combination of hand and mouth, and obviously no teeth. The other thing, so far as style and technique goes, is that it's another thing you learn with each other. Little details, learn what your partner likes. I remember being with this girl once when we were in Spain and this girl started yanking on my dick like it was made out of steel and I didn't know how to say slow or soft in Spanish. So the next day, I was going to see the girl again and I learned 'despacio' means slowly and 'lento' means soft, so I was like, 'Lento, lento!'

JESSE HUGHES: I sum up the best technique for a blowjob like this: by describing my worst blowjob ever. It was amazing!

JIMMY ASHHURST: I've never really known what was going on down there. It's hard to tell if they're using any particular skill or whether their mouth is just sort of open. I've been able to tell the good ones from the bad ones and there is definitely a large spectrum of that going on. I think a lot of it has to do with the circumstances, but some of them try and get a little too tricky; I mean, it's not rocket science… I can imagine; I wouldn't know.

LEMMY: No, I don't think so. I think I'm afraid I'm going to come up with the same thing again – it's always personal. Some chicks like one thing, some chicks like another. Straight on the thing is good. I mean, they always seem to like that, as I do too.

NICKE BORG: To be really honest, I've never ever been a 'give me a blowjob' kind of guy. I think it's over-rated. Maybe it's just me, I don't know. But sometimes, you get very, very surprised. I guess most people are doing it the wrong way, so that's not what I really find to be the most wow. So for me, I wouldn't even know the best technique. Go slow! 'Give it time. I've done a gram of coke for fuck's sake, take it easy.'

ROB PATTERSON: Nah, I'm easy.

TOBY RAND: It's when a girl puts her tongue around the top of your cock and rings it 'round.

VAZQUEZ: For me, I'm not really nuts about getting head. But there are two women that come to mind from the past. There was this one who could actually get it into her throat and that was like, 'Holy shit! I thought that was just a myth.' That was pretty crazy.

Does hot or cold turn people on more?

ACEY SLADE: I like to be in control, so I'm usually the one initiating that. I get a little freaked out when a girl uses a hot or cold thing because that usually means I'm not the one holding the reins.

ADDE: That's just for having fun with it; it doesn't have anything to do with sex… like putting ice in your mouth, or putting hot chocolate in your mouth. It's just the fun part of it; it has nothing to do with sex.

BRENT MUSCAT: I had a girl chew ice one time and she had ice in her mouth. I didn't think it was a big deal either way.

CHIP Z'NUFF: I'm told the ice cube trick is pretty good. Like Karma Sutra, where you can put the ice cube on certain parts of the body and then go from putting an ice cube on it to putting your mouth on it. However, I haven't really tried it.

DANKO JONES: I've tried that shit and it's just very distracting for me.

JESSE HUGHES: To me, the exotic acutrama normally is context. If you happen to be in the kitchen and you bust out the ice-creams, it's freaky shit.

JIMMY ASHHURST: I like the hotter things myself.

ROB PATTERSON: Like temperature? Hot, definitely hot.

CANDLE WAX IS SUCH A CLICHÉ BUT IT'S FUCKING EXCITING WHAT YOU CAN DO WITH IT.

TOBY RAND: I love using ice – love it. I love having it used on me. Cold fruit, whatever it is, just whatever tastes good. Definitely cold stuff turns me on because you're obviously already hot. Candle wax is such a cliché but it's fucking exciting what you can do with it. So let's put both down.

VAZQUEZ: As long as the mouth is there, I'll take room temperature.

What's the best way to get erect again as fast as possible after an orgasm?

ACEY SLADE: One of the gifts of sobriety is that this hasn't been an issue to me. Starting foreplay again with the girl is definitely going to arouse you again – start the vicious cycle all over again.

ANDREW W.K.: Probably oral sex; I think so. It depends on maybe also taking a very brief nap; a very short nap of like 20 minutes to let your body reset. You wake up and it can seem like it's been a really long time. It also really helps if the girl is really, really, really beautiful.

BLASKO: It kind of just happens. Like, some people are built that way and some people aren't. I don't know if there's any sort of technique. I'm sort of blessed with the first part in the sense that I don't really have an issue with it, so it doesn't really take much effort.

CHIP Z'NUFF: Wait 15 to 20 minutes and then dine on her. If you're doing that, that will get you excited one more time. You'll be able to have at least a couple of rounds.

DOUG ROBB: Blowjobs. I think that's unanimous, c'mon!

HANDSOME DICK MANITOBA: Usually boobs turn me on. Boobs for me is usually a surefire way. Grabbing boobs or playing with boobs and having the girl really into it, grabbing me and going, 'C'mon, c'mon!' Just being really into it. But usually I just like to relax for a while after the first one. It's a mental thing. I guess when I was younger I was driven more to do it again as quick as possible, but now it's more about the long… instead of doing it and coming and doing it again, I'd rather have a long experience and then come and be done. That's been my MO lately.

JESSE HUGHES: The best way to get erect again after an orgasm, because as you all know, the penis loses 70% of its blood after orgasm… the best way to achieve an erection immediately after is to really be into chicks still, after you come.

JIMMY ASHHURST: Change partners.

LEMMY: I don't know mate. The cattle prod springs to mind. Sometimes you're lucky; sometimes you're not.

ROB PATTERSON: Wait five minutes.

TOBY RAND: Headjob – it's a one word answer.

VAZQUEZ: For me, it's just like I'll start fingering my girl and she'll start flipping out and shit, and then all of a sudden I'm on my back.

What's the best way to stimulate a clitoris with your mouth?

ACEY SLADE: Just find the little man in the canoe and make little circles around him.

ADDE: Do the alphabet!

ALLISON ROBERTSON: It's really hard to give pointers to be honest. I just think that's the kind of thing you have to know the other person's preferences completely because I've never heard anyone agree on that. I've heard so many different things from girlfriends that vary from what I like or whatever. Then you get guys who are like, 'Well I did this and this with this girlfriend and she liked it. Why don't you?' Everybody's completely different, you know? To me, it's not about skill and more about figuring it out with the person. There are a lot of ways and a lot of people think they're Don Juan and stuff, but there's just no right answer.

ANDREW W.K.: The tongue for sure, but more specifically with that, thinking of the tongue as a finger in itself, one that has an infinite number of knuckles like a snake and being really consistent yet varied, if that makes any sense. When you start with something, you've got to stick with it for a while. It's like a patient approach, but you can never zone out. You can't lose your awareness; you've got to be really present but always stick with a move a little bit longer than you think you should, so just when you think, 'OK, I've been doing this move long enough,' then think, 'OK, now I'm really starting with it.'

BLASKO: That's too hard to describe verbally.

BRENT MUSCAT: Just kind of suck on it a little bit. Put your mouth on it and wiggle your tongue a little bit.

CHIP Z'NUFF: With your mouth, just gently up and down. There's no reason to go back and forth like a jag-off. Just up and down, nice and slow and then with the two fingers in there playing bass. That whole technique together. I wrote the book on that. It's called *Playing Bass* by Chip Z'Nuff.

COURTNEY TAYLOR-TAYLOR: Just anything very, very lightly.

DANKO JONES: Well I've been told I have a long tongue and I think I do. My technique is to stick out my tongue and make sure it goes from the top to the bottom and then you just slap it on like a piece of meat and you very, very gently move it around. They don't get a licking sensation but just this overall blanketed feeling. So I just put my tongue against them and very gently curl it or wave it; that always works well. The licking is great too and Sam Kinison always said, and I have put his advice into action so I know it works, and he said just lick the alphabet. That way, the girl gets a different sensation and also you have to listen to whenever she really gets turned-on by her breathing or whatever comes out of her mouth, then you follow that up. You don't do it too much; you have to change it up a bit subtly.

DOUG ROBB: I would say kind of suck on it and at the same time tickle it with your tongue.

GINGER: Use the tongue, not too softly but definitely not too hard; plenty of saliva. Ron Jeremy recommends you trace letters of the alphabet on the clitoris, and I have to say it works a treat. Be consistent with your rhythm. You want to feel her every move and not bring her to climax too early. Always ask her to tell you when you're doing it perfectly.

HANDSOME DICK MANITOBA: The best advice I ever got was from talking to a lesbian. She said, 'You know how much attention you take to kissing, trying to be a good kisser and grabbing the moment and being relaxed with your tongue as the absolute appetiser of the sexual experience? If you get down there, it's just like another mouth. Get lost in it and just treat it like it's another mouth.' I find that isolating the clitoris and lightly teasing it with your tongue... basically most girls like the same thing but there are different details; every human being is not exactly the same. So you can tell by the writhing, by the sounds and by the motion that you're headed in the right direction; you're on the right road. Like a dick touch: too hard, too soft, a little lighter with this. There are different parts of the sexual experience that leads you to, 'All right, touch me a little harder now.' I find nice, soft caressing and following the lead is best. You'll get your working orders as you're going along.

JESSE HUGHES: I find that girls in general are appreciative when you in any way enthusiastically go down without requiring prodding. I simply use the tongue and use it in whatever direction until I hear them doing the thing that lets me know they like it. Normally they say something like, 'I like it.'

JIMMY ASHHURST: That is rocket science. I will never know. Just try everything man. Somebody has said lick the alphabet and when you end up at a certain letter she makes a noise or something. That's still a mystery, but I don't think it's meant to be figured out, you know? We have a lifetime, so try everything you can.

JOEL O'KEEFFE: Lip-sync all the words to your favourite song on her sex-fuelled jukebox. If you can't think of anything, try 'Walk This Way' by Aerosmith for its fast verse vocals and fat choruses – but you've got to mimic the big Steve Tyler lip movements to get the full effect. If you can do all that, it will drive her crazy!

LEMMY: Side to side. That's the way they do it.

NICKE BORG: Go easy. Let it accelerate. Look at the face; how is she reacting? Does she look like she's fucking really enjoying it? Is she shaking? How's she feeling; is she warm, cold? Go very, very slow and work your way.

ROB PATTERSON: Well, I have a tongue piercing – do the math.

TOBY RAND: I actually like to make out with it like I'm making out with their actual mouth. So I kiss them down there like I kiss them on their mouth. A girl will know that when she makes out with me that's what she's going to get downstairs and from there they can tell me what else they want. I love direction – love it!

VAZQUEZ: You've got to ask the woman what she wants. Some want it real gentle like your tongue's a fucking feather. Some women want you to suck it like you're going to give it a God-damn hickey! So I always ask the women what they want.

How do you influence the taste or volume of your semen?

ACEY SLADE: I've never tasted my cum. I'm picturing these guys who say you can change the taste of it. I'm picturing them having like a bunch of Dixie Cups lined up at their house and having a clothes peg on their nose, wearing one of those sterile nuclear outfits, sitting there sticking their tongue in these little Dixie Cups saying, 'Oh God that was gross, but I think it does taste like pineapple!

BLASKO: I don't know that you can. I know that some people have said celery. I tried it and didn't really notice much of a difference. I think some people are just born that way.

CHIP Z'NUFF: One of the big porn stars told me great advice: to have good tasting cum would be to drink a lot of pineapple juice and eat tons of celery. The celery will give you a rig like Chinese Arithmetic, so I recommend raw celery sticks (it's really good for you) and pineapple juice. Don't drink a lot of coffee. Xaviera Hollander in the book *The Happy Hooker* recommends you don't eat a lot of candies and don't drink a lot of coffee. Men that drink tons of coffee and eat tons of chocolates and candy have terrible tasting cum.

TO HAVE GOOD TASTING CUM WOULD BE TO DRINK A LOT OF PINEAPPLE JUICE AND EAT TONS OF CELERY

DANKO JONES: I guess don't jerk off for a while, but in terms of diet I always heard that zinc works and tuna – that's what I heard.

JESSE HUGHES: I've heard lettuce.

JIMMY ASHHURST: I've heard things about vodka, grapefruit juice… I've never really been one for planning ahead, so it's sort of hard to think about that. Like, 'I'd better drink some fucking grapefruit juice.' Who does that?

NICKE BORG: There's a stand-up comedy guy that I know well and… do you know that coconut chocolate bar called Bounty? Well, he once greased himself in fucking coconut milk or something and the chick was like, 'What have you done, did you eat a Bounty?' Ha! But when it comes to cum, don't let it be in there for too many days. The bass player from my friend's band once told his girlfriend the reason why he jerks off – because she was kind of disappointed, like, 'Don't you think that I'm…' – so he was like, 'Well if you don't jerk off like twice a day, your semen will rot in your body!' So, old semen – if you haven't had an ejaculation for a long time – your semen will taste like shit. Don't do it like ten times before you fuck, but don't let it be for like two weeks before you have sex with your girl or then your cum will taste bad – it'll be rotten basically, according to what this bass player says.

ROB PATTERSON: Grapefruit juice, or is that a wives' tale?

TOBY RAND: Celery! Without a doubt, mate – it's amazing! That's my best tip. Eat bunches of it, as much as you can, and you'll cum in glorious bucket loads. The chicks love it! Ask her [points to his current blonde actress girlfriend]… she's smiling, right?

VAZQUEZ: I've never really tried that. I've heard that you can eat a bunch of celery or something and shoot like loads and loads, but I wouldn't really want to do that. I'm Latin; I'm already too fertile to begin with.

ROMANCING & WINNING HEARTS

"THE HEART OF ROMANCE IS SIMPLY BEING ATTENTIVE. TEND TO YOUR LOVER. PAY ATTENTION TO YOUR LOVER"

What's the best way to someone's heart?

ACEY SLADE: For me, probably a sense of humour and a feeling of stability. For me, if I'm with someone who can give me a feeling of stability, that's the biggest thing. If I don't feel stable and I don't feel safe… us musicians, we're unstable people. I know I can bring stability to a relationship; for a musician, I do really good. I can pay the bills, I can take care of everything if I have to, but then it still comes down to the emotional security. With my ex-wife, I paid for everything and kept a roof over our head and everything, but the emotional stability wasn't there and that's really what's needed.

ALLISON ROBERTSON: I think listening to them and listening to what they say and not just trying to constantly impress them or talk about yourself or even just being hot all the time as a girl. I think it's more important to be like a friend and listen to them, because at the end of the day, to me, it seems that most of my boyfriends have appreciated that I have good advice or just listen to them when they need to talk. Men, you know, they don't always talk to each other about what's on their mind, so they need a confidante and, as a woman, that's a nice thing to be.

BLASKO: I think honesty is probably the best way to their heart.

BRENT MUSCAT: Being around and spending a lot of time. Talking a lot and finding things in common I think is the best way. If you like the same band, maybe you could take her to the concert and listen to the music together. Find out what they like too. Like I said, a lot of sex is really in between your ears, in your brain. A lot of it is just finding common ground and finding the connection that way.

CHIP Z'NUFF: Through her stomach. Women love to eat. Take her out to a great dinner or you cook a great dinner for her. You don't even have to take her out to eat, just bring her to your pad and cook a great dinner for her, like Adler's stroganoff. Immediately, you're a happy guy. Great food is a great barometer for getting the ball rolling and shows the kind of character you have too.

COURTNEY TAYLOR-TAYLOR: Just be easy-going; strong enough to just be easy-going.

DANKO JONES: Being very honest, upfront, with no drama, no bullshit and make her laugh.

DOUG ROBB: Humour. I think guys with a good sense of humour and guys who don't take themselves too seriously at all moments – at some points you have to take yourself seriously, but I think if you kind of take life as it goes and are not so highly strung about everything... I could be totally wrong, but I kind of feel that girls appreciate that; a guy who can laugh at himself.

JAMES KOTTAK: A beautiful song, a bouquet of flowers and some great food.

JESSE HUGHES: This is actually my favourite topic because romance is the coolest thing in the world. It really is and an unfortunate side-effect of rock'n'roll and pop culture was a loss of the romantic side of the love equation. Romance is the most beautiful thing. The best way to a woman's heart is simply by observing that woman. That's more of a philosophy instead of a specific way, but everything's situational and girls are the same way; they're situational and so context is king. The heart of romance is simply being attentive. Tend to your lover. Pay attention to your lover. When you're watching them a little more deeply than simply kissing ass, you'll notice certain things and then romance is simply a demonstration that you've paid attention to something deeper than the flesh.

JIMMY ASHHURST: Security: I think all women are looking for that in the end.

LEMMY: Make her laugh. Tell her a joke or two. Crack her up; that'll get it.

ROB PATTERSON: For me it's brains and self-confidence.

TOBY RAND: Confident honesty, where someone is not afraid to be who they are and they're not afraid to show you affection or show you bits about them. My experiences have been that you meet people who are so fake and you just long for someone who's just honest and cool and chilled. I think that a chilled girl, who's relaxed with herself and just rad and wants to do whatever; it's the biggest turn-on and way to my heart.

VAZQUEZ: Obviously you've got to talk to them, and you've got to listen – at least you've got to pretend. I think a lot of it has got to do with chemistry. My Dad has always said to me, 'You know, people say sex isn't everything, but if you can't get that right with a woman, the whole thing is going to go to fucking shit.' You have to have that chemistry; you've got to be able to talk to them. They've got to know that you understand.

How can you show your partner that you are truly in love with them?

ACEY SLADE: For me, the way that I was showing my ex that I loved her was telling her about tours that I had coming up and how much they were going to pay, making her feel like she was a part of what was going on, because I've always been really selfish with my career and with my music. Let's face it, success is an elusive thing and I've always had the attitude of, 'There's a tour up; I've got to do it. I don't care if I don't make this much money or that much money. It doesn't matter if your mum's going to be here on vacation, whatever.' Like, that's the way I've always been. So I think to me, showing love was like saying, 'Hey, this is the opportunity I have. What do you think?'

ADDE: I'd tell her all the time that I love her and I appreciate her. I'd just give her all the love that I've got.

ALLISON ROBERTSON: I feel like when someone can really trust the other one. It's when you can tell that they're not looking at anyone else or thinking about anyone else. That to me is like the ultimate. I'm in a band and I see a lot of people around. There are a lot of cute guys, a lot of stupid guys, and plenty of people trying to hit on me, but I think a guy knows when I'm either in love or just care about that particular guy because I completely ignore the advances of all the other people. That's like an ultimate sacrifice for a guy, so I don't expect it as quickly from a man. Some guys just like to look around and I think that's OK too – with no touchy.

ANDREW W.K.: I think really letting them be. Being unconditionally supportive and completely open-minded and letting them fully flourish and revel in doing what they want to do. It's letting someone go and being very detached while also being as un-detached as you can possibly be. I think that's really a balance when you have enough confidence in yourself that you can fully unleash that confidence in the other person. I think that's when you're in the best state of love.

BLASKO: Listen to them.

BRENT MUSCAT: Being kind to them and spending a lot of time with them. Taking them places and I guess telling them, 'Hey, I've really grown attached to you and I love you.' Tell them that you love them.

CHIP Z'NUFF: Oh actions speak louder than words, and not just buying gifts for them, just by spending time and listening to them speak and doing little small things for them. I don't care if it's taking the garbage out, to doing laundry and hanging up clothes, making the bed. Just small little things sometimes trip the girl's trigger. They say, 'Wow, I'm not used to this.' Opening the car door is very respectful. Anything gentlemanly usually wins.

DANKO JONES: In this line of work, you have to reassure and then reassure again. That's with someone who is secure with themselves and who isn't needy. Then after you do that, they've just got to trust you. So I just reassure them by being truthful, showing them that I'm truthful in other areas of my life, not necessarily about women and cheating, just about what I like and being very consistent with the food I like or a shirt I like. Anything as small as that reassures them that, 'Yeah, he is consistent with what he says.' That's very important if you want to be in a serious relationship with someone and tour playing rock'n'roll music, etc, etc. You've got to do that. Also, another thing I found is introducing her to your friends and your family – if you show me who your friends are, I'll tell you who you are. If you introduce her to your friend who does bong hits all day and scours the classifieds for hookers, carries a shotgun and has a nice gun collection going at home and deals blow on the side, then she might start thinking, 'Well maybe this guy...' You don't show her that friend! You show her the nice friend. So for someone in a band, I think that's what you should do; show them your nice, stable friends, the normal friends that you have, and be consistent with what you say and always be honest. That's how you build her trust and eventually you can leave and go on tour and there won't be any neediness from her or any insecurities. You won't have to deal with her crying on the phone before you go onstage because she heard something from someone or some fucking bullshit like that and you take care of it.

DOUG ROBB: By sacrificing things that you love to do, to do stuff with them, without them asking.

HANDSOME DICK MANITOBA: I just respect them. I think one of the hardest things of being in a relationship and being very, very close to someone – and this goes for *any* relationship, it doesn't have to be romantic – is that they're not you. That's hard to take sometimes. They're not you, they don't have to have your feelings, or share this or share that. They're them and even if it's completely different, it's just accepting them. It's who they are. You want to come together and be together; that's your choice. Loving them is loving them; it's accepting them for who they are – not who you can mould them into – and respecting them for who they are.

JAMES KOTTAK: When they're totally sick and throwing up and you sit there, instead of going for a night out in Hollywood, you sit there and you help clean up the puke.

JIMMY ASHHURST: If you're prepared to take a stab at offering them security that would be a good indication.

LEMMY: Cut out your heart and offer it to them.

ROB PATTERSON: Love is felt, not shown.

TOBY RAND: When you're with your partner, you just want to be with them the whole time. When you're not with them, you know that moment when you see them for the first time and you have that look in your eyes and you just want to grab them – I think that's more than any materialistic kind of crap.

VAZQUEZ: I suppose you could write them a song. You write them a song and then sing it to them and it's like – bam! It doesn't have to be like 'Baby, I Love Your Way' – it doesn't have to be that good. The fact that you made it for them and it's theirs, they love that man.

What's the most romantic thing someone has done for you?

ACEY SLADE: Honestly, I had a girl that I was dating; we'd been dating for a while when one day, out of the blue, she just showed up with roses, for no reason.

ADDE: Going on a long trip just to see me, for like 12 hours, and then go right back because I'm just going on tour. That's really romantic.

ALLISON ROBERTSON: I think that would be listening to me and actually letting me be myself. To me, that's the most romantic. It's not even a gesture; it's more like an all-round thing that doesn't happen very often where someone actually listens to you and remembers what you said. Recently, somebody's been really listening to me a lot. He ordered food for me and remembered what I eat at this particular place (I'm a vegetarian). I'm more impressed with someone that's thoughtful than like who spends money or does a bunch of grandiose things. To me, I'm more impressed when somebody actually listens to what you had to say and remembered it and then applied it later.

BRUCE KULICK: On occasion I've gotten a gift that I've thought was ultra-perfect for me and I'm really hard to get gifts for because I've been fortunate; I know what I like and I buy what I like. I treat myself all the time and then usually when people buy me something it's something I don't want. So when I've got a gift that I sorely needed but I was either too lazy or too shy to make the purchase that means a lot to me. It could be something as silly as a digital camera and a movie that I've been dying to see. I guess it's that old saying, 'Do unto others as you want people to do for you', so I think any time in my life that I've had someone make an effort for me... I'll give you one that doesn't work: my ex-wife thought it would be a lot of fun to rent a vintage car on my birthday to drive. I like cars; I'm not a car freak though. It's kind of cool to drive an old Cadillac, but not when it's stalling in the middle of traffic and it's just a noisy gas-guzzling beast. So her intention was good but it didn't work out and I actually really hated my gift. So be careful: if you're going to do an extreme gift for somebody, be sure that it's absolutely what they want – that goes a long way.

CHIP Z'NUFF: I guess the most romantic thing anybody's ever done for me is my first wife gave me a beautiful baby daughter. That was the most romantic thing ever; a daughter named Tara. She's now 24. Out of everything and all the people I've spent quality time with, that was the most romantic thing. I've had nice things given to me and I've spent quality time with beautiful goddesses, but that's the one that stands out – just a beautiful little girl. It changes you. You can tell right away. It's a piece of you and it's a blessing.

COURTNEY TAYLOR-TAYLOR: Taking care of me when I'm ill.

DANKO JONES: I guess flying in to see me for one night and then flying back.

DOUG ROBB: Saying yes when I asked her to propose. Maybe I've got a terrible memory, but that's the only thing that comes to mind. I was just glad she didn't say no.

HANDSOME DICK MANITOBA: I'd have to go back to the best 'I love you' that I ever heard, which was when my girl Zoe was having a Caesarean and I'm basically sitting there holding her torso, holding her hand. I'm like hanging out with her torso while the doctors are working with the lower-half of her body behind the curtain. We're waiting for our son and I'm almost 49 years old, waiting for my first kid in my life. They come around the curtain and hand me this little gorgeous bundle of baby boy and they go, 'This is your son' and I completely fucking turn to mush and Zoe looked at me and went, 'I love you.' It was like the purest moment of 'I love you'. The greatest 'I love you' I ever heard.

JAMES KOTTAK: Pulled my head out of the toilet when I was barfing.

SHE HAD AN ADOLF HITLER DOLL, TWO CANDLES AND A BOTTLE OF SPARKLING APPLE JUICE WAITING FOR ME ON MY BIRTHDAY.

JESSE HUGHES: I dated a girl who was Chinese (and I only mention that because she was a sort of Asian, Mata Hari, assassin, cold-blooded person) and she was a reporter for the *Naked News*. We dated very, very seriously and she used to call me The Happy Dictator and all this jazz and she was independently wealthy. She went onto some website and paid five grand for a 12-inch doll that was a meticulous re-creation of Adolf Hitler, with two uniforms. She had an Adolf Hitler doll, two candles and a bottle of sparkling apple juice (because I don't drink) waiting for me on my birthday. I couldn't tell if I should be turned on like, 'You vill do it' Gestapo-style or if I should be totally insulted. It was the most bizarrely romantic situation. There was nothing cool about Hitler. I want to make the T-shirt that says, 'Hitler – What an Asshole!' So, you give that as a gift and you are Asian; that's really weird, for sure.

JIMMY ASHHURST: Making brownies and making a book called What I Love About You, where they just entered a bunch of little things… must have friggin' taken them forever.

LEMMY: I once got a voodoo doll put through my letterbox in London with a load of pins in the genitals. I must have done something wrong to somebody, right? Or it could have been from her boyfriend, I suppose.

NICKE BORG: Appreciating me the way that I am. Telling me that it's OK. Telling me, 'I don't really want you to do that but it's OK because you will eventually find out that you don't want to do that to yourself anyway. But it's OK because I love you.' So basically, just understanding – like totally fucking dedicating your life to someone. That's the most romantic thing, I think.

ROB PATTERSON: My fiancée showed up in Germany when I was on tour on Valentine's Day and decorated the hotel room with all kinds of stuff when I left for a few minutes. It was so damn cute.

TOBY RAND: I was playing a show and I thought that person wasn't in the country and she had avoided my phone calls just so she could keep her story up, and then I looked out in the audience and she was sitting in the audience.

VAZQUEZ: I have this ex-girlfriend who made this book for me of like artwork and all this poetry and shit, and pictures of us and everything. It was really fucking moving; it was nice. I really dug that a lot.

What gift best says 'I love you'?

ACEY SLADE: I used to think it was guitars, then I thought it was tattoos. Giving themselves unconditionally. I know it sounds corny. I've dated women who have a lot of money that will buy you things and that can be a trap too; that's no good. So I think it's just giving themselves.

ALLISON ROBERTSON: Flowers... I'm just kidding! For me, I like presents. So if there's something I've been talking about, it's always nice if someone gets it for you, but to be honest I really think something like cooking dinner or making me something from scratch is more of an 'I love you' kind of thing than a present. Also, I think taking a trip is a nice present, saying, 'Hey, we're going here and we're doing this', because I don't really get to take trips for fun. I'm always travelling but it's not really fun – it's fun but it's not relaxed, because I'm still working.

ANDREW W.K.: Something very thoughtful, usually. The ones I've thought were most thoughtful, whether they were fancy or very modest in their monetary value, it's how it related to some aspect of my life that was unique and only this person, this woman, could be familiar with. Whether it's a little piece of equipment for my studio, whether it's some food item, whether it's something around the house, those very thoughtful ones to me say the most.

BLASKO: I think sex. I think that'll get the job done.

BRENT MUSCAT: Jewellery is good because it lasts usually forever, where something like a rose is dead in a few days and looks ugly. So jewellery would be nice. Something they could wear and think about you. A ring or necklace would be good.

CHIP Z'NUFF: Actions. Your actions – that's the gift. She's still going to get mad at you if you come home late. She's still going to be pissed off at you if she's got the beautiful mansion and you're not there. So the gift of kindness and being nice is best. Spend quality time with them. That's what we all want. You see an old couple out there and they're holding hands and hanging out together, that's what everybody else is looking for if you think about it. I hail that! There's nothing like seeing an old couple walking down the street. It's so charming and it's real. It's not contrived. It's very organic and there's nothing like it.

COURTNEY TAYLOR-TAYLOR: A weekend at the beach with a hot tub in the room. Just getting away from everybody else with someone.

DANKO JONES: I really suck at gifts.

DOUG ROBB: Time. I think spending time and having undivided attention is worth more than anything you can buy. In my case, it feels that way because I'm gone so much that time spent together is invaluable.

GINGER: Something novel that you think she'll like. Even if she doesn't she will still appreciate the thought that has gone into it. Flowers are lame, chocolates are a no-no and teddy bears could make her think you see her as a child. There's no need to spend a lot, but if you do see something costly that reminds you of her then it's only money and you're more likely to make it back if you have love in your life.

JAMES KOTTAK: I would have to say a nice Mercedes E430 isn't bad.

JESSE HUGHES: Diamonds are a girl's best friend. Gentlemen prefer blondes, but blondes don't like cripples. So with that being said, it depends, man. The most romantic gift you can give someone is a gift that demonstrates you are paying attention, but also classic silly things, corniness and clichés could be the most useful, romantic gift. What I mean by that is: you're at a restaurant and you have a special little desert brought over with a candle and a couple of the maître d's come by and clap for no reason. Also, not just giving gifts but the moment of when you give the gift. Giving the gift on an off occasion when there is no occasion at all to get it; not on Valentine's Day, but on a day that has nothing attached to it is when you score the biggest rock points! And giving the gift in front of a remote audience that you are not present at; ie mail flowers.

JIMMY ASHHURST: Anything in a Tiffany's box, man.

LEMMY: Diamonds.

NICKE BORG: To really, really make your loved one understand and believe that you are actually caring and there for that person. Especially in really hard and difficult times, if you just show that you are actually there as a support, it can be the best gift. I'm not that much into presents. Everybody appreciates flowers – that's always nice – but talking about *really* giving your loved one a gift is that you're there for them when they fucking need it.

ROB PATTERSON: A Pro-Tools rig? Ha.

TOBY RAND: A bottle of Jägermeister… and sitting on the couch drinking it together. A bottle of anything with two glasses.

VAZQUEZ: Honestly, I don't think gifts do it, man.

SAFE SEX
(CONTRACEPTIVES & STDS)

"I WILL ONLY HAVE SEX WITHOUT A CONDOM IF I THINK I HAVE A FUTURE WITH THE PERSON"

What is the most important safety precaution to take?

ACEY SLADE: Definitely a condom; 100% a condom.

ADDE: I'm so horrible with that because as soon as I get drunk and I find a girl, we end up in bed and I don't want to wear a rubber and when I'm drunk it's like, 'I don't care if I get something in my system!', so I'm horrible with that – horrible.

ALLISON ROBERTSON: A condom, for sure.

BLASKO: The safest thing to do is to not do it at all. Short of that, wear a condom.

BRENT MUSCAT: A condom is always good. I think if you're active, you should probably go to the doctor at least every six months and get a check-up. And be clean; be aware of your body. Shower every day and look at yourself. Be aware of what's going on. If something's not normal with you, you should go to the doctor and check it out. Definitely don't have sex if something's going on. Use condoms as much as you can.

STAY OFF THE BLOW, A LITTLE BIT, UNTIL YOU GET THE CONDOM ON, AND THEN YOU DO A LINE - AND THEN YOU FUCK.

BRUCE KULICK: Well of course wearing a condom, and if you're in a committed relationship that's not important, but when you're not I think it's imperative. It's always been very easy for me to wear a condom and I was always very careful. There's no little Bruces that I know of out there.

CHIP Z'NUFF: For sure, you have to have a Trojan. You have to have some kind of protection on the guy. They have things for girls now, too. Let me tell you: I don't like any of that stuff because it takes all the romance out. If you're going to be a guy who's real promiscuous or if you're with a woman who you feel is promiscuous, make sure you wear something. But if it's just your chick and stuff, you don't need to have that kind of stuff I don't think. I think you're better off just being careful. Make sure that before you get ready to come, you take out. Don't come inside, because then you've got to worry about that for the next 30 days as to what's going to happen. So my recommendation is prophylactic and if it's a girl and they think it's questionable, they've got it for girls too. Don't wear more than one; just wear one. Don't put two rubbers on for that girl. No, that doesn't do any good. It's terrible. Ask any doctor and he'll tell you two rubbers is a joke. It's a fallacy and it doesn't work. Just one good rubber and just be careful. For the woman, after she's done having sex, I recommend her to go right to the bathroom and she can clean herself out. She then has a better chance of being safe.

DANKO JONES: Well you've got to wear a condom; I guess that would be the first thing. Also being very choosy and picky. From my perspective, from a guy in a band's perspective (unless you're playing in a black metal band), chances are if you're playing rock'n'roll after a few years you've been able to meet a lot of girls that you wouldn't have met if you work at the bank. So over the years of meeting these girls and everything, you kind of develop a sixth sense. So you should use a lot of discretion that you've learned, that you've honed from your experience on the road. It just comes with experience where I can now look at someone and go, 'Drama! Get me away from her!'

DOUG ROBB: Condoms.

EVAN SEINFELD: In the adult industry we have a strict testing policy where we have an upscale, full-panel screening, but guys – wear a condom.

JAMES KOTTAK: Don't do it. When in doubt, kick 'em out.

JESSE HUGHES: The most important safety precaution to take during sex is not dying.

JIMMY ASHHURST: A condom – absolutely.

LEMMY: Have a gun under the pillow – that's the safest.

NICKE BORG: Nobody wants to have a disease and these days we have diseases that are lethal. And I'm not very proud of myself for having non-protected sex many, many times with people who really could have had whatever. A condom is a condom, so just try to fucking use condoms and try to make something sexy about it. Of course, everybody agrees that it's not as nice having fucking rubber around your dick – fine. Stay off the blow, a little bit, until you get the condom on, and then you do a line – and then you fuck.

ROB PATTERSON: Condoms.

TOBY RAND: The most important safety precaution is if you wear a condom. Actually, the safest precaution is not to have sex at all... just get blowjobs.

VAZQUEZ: Keep the fucking lights on, OK? You want to see what the fuck is going on. Obviously, you've got to use condoms man, I mean, what the fuck? But keep the lights on or you don't know what the fuck you're getting into.

How can you be confident you're not going to catch anything before engaging with a partner?

ACEY SLADE: I think by just using common sense; look at the person. I've turned down sex with girls before that were really attractive. They knew the tour manager and name-dropped a bunch of bands and you really have to think about that – is it worth dying for? You always have to use a condom though. It doesn't stop you from having sex on tour; nothing's going to stop that, but it can come close.

ALLISON ROBERTSON: I'm a really safe kind of person so I usually have to trust them, but you can never be sure. That's why you have to take precautions. You can feel secure but you might not find out about something until later. I think you can hope for the best but in the meantime you have to use a condom.

ANDREW W.K.: I guess to ask and talk about it. Say, 'I don't have this' or 'I do have this' or whatever and ask for them to do the same thing. It's interesting because my Dad and other people that have been much older than me say that they feel so bad for me because when they were my age no one thought about that stuff and no one had to worry about it. I wonder if that's because it didn't exist or if they just didn't think about it. I imagine that, maybe not AIDS or HIV for example, but pretty much the whole other gamut of diseases was out there; it just doesn't seem as people were as educated. My generation and every one since has had a really heavy dose of sexual education, specifically on safe sex and wearing condoms and all these awful diseases that were just described in the most acute detail, with every discharge described in colour and taste and smell and consistency. It was really horrifying and they made extreme efforts to make sex and the diseases you could get as disgusting and repulsive as they could. And that really worked! For me, I avoided a lot of sexual experience, sometimes just out of fear of getting some awful disease. So since then, talking with people and trying to have them be really honest is the best defence. But even then, there have been girls who have lied and I found out sometimes months and months and months later that they had some disease. Asking them is really the only solution; otherwise you're taking a risk each time.

COURTNEY TAYLOR-TAYLOR: You can't. You just have to be with the same person.

DANKO JONES: Yeah, that's crazy. First of all, look for cold sores, then a certain amount of talking and getting to know the person I suppose. It's only one night a lot of the time, so it's hard to say. Condom wearing is supposed to be the almost sure thing.

HANDSOME DICK MANITOBA: You really can't. You've got to use protection, but you really can't because there's genetic history, a blood history. There's a moment that happens where everyone has a few drinks in them and you're about to lie down with somebody you don't know, and you can't ask her for her medical chart, so you protect yourself as best as possible. That's one of the toughest things in life that I think about having to tell my kid about. That moment comes and you get so out of your mind as the hormones take over and just thrust you forward into the situation and you don't care any more about anything except the moment and then you wind up paying for it for a lifetime. I grew up in a different era where, if anything went wrong, you might have to go and get some medicine or some pills, but you'll be OK. Then the era of AIDS came along and now you can die from sex, so there are different things kids are growing up with. You can be as safe as possible, but like I say, you can't ask for any medical history.

JESSE HUGHES: Don't have sex with a catcher's mit. You know what? You pretty much are what you eat and the same thing's true with sex. If you're Dorothy and you land in Hollywood, then it's junkies and hookers and queers. But I say if you get AIDS, make lemonades.

JIMMY ASHHURST: You can never be entirely comfortable. That's when things start to go awry.

LEMMY: Don't fuck anybody. The condom protects you against most diseases, right?

TOBY RAND: I think in this day and age, no one can ever be really comfortable unless you actually have an STD test right in front of you – it's getting that way.

VAZQUEZ: Obviously you use condoms and shit, but it's all a fucking gamble. It's like, who the fuck knows?

What is the best thing to do if you don't have any condoms available?

ACEY SLADE: Then you don't have sex. I watched a friend of mine's brother die from AIDS and it's the most undignified way to die unfortunately. I'm thankful that I had that experience. I went for four years of having sex, while being in a relationship, and being like, 'No, we need to use a condom.' One thing that's totally fucked up that a lot of band guys do is they're in relationships where they have a wife or a girlfriend back home and they fuck around on the road without a condom. That is so irresponsible and fucked up! It's bad enough that you're playing emotional games. So when you're doing that, you're saying you're not 100% into the relationship but the other person doesn't know that; they're just an innocent victim. So then if you give them something they have to have for the rest of their life because you weren't 100% committed, then that's not fair.

ADDE: I would probably take it off anyway, so…

ALLISON ROBERTSON: Go get some! I really think in this world, you just have to have them. I think guys should definitely have them. Not that I wouldn't buy them or anything, but I always spend a lot of money on other things. I think that's the guy's responsibility.

ANDREW W.K.: Everything you can do without making contact with a mucous membrane, so that's basically going to be hands, and you can get a little detached at that point.

BLASKO: Oral sex.

BRENT MUSCAT: Go buy some. There are condoms everywhere nowadays; they're in every convenience store. I remember I was dating a girl and I would go to her house. This was probably 10 years ago when I was living in LA. I'd always go, 'Shit! I don't have condoms.' She'd say, 'Well let's go to your car and go to the store' and it's kind of exciting. You might have to wait a few minutes but at least you know for sure you're going to get laid. If she's telling you to go to the store to get condoms you know you're in. But that's the best thing I think – a lot of clubs have them in the bathroom, bathroom attendants usually have them, or friends. Most people have them on them.

BRUCE KULICK: Oh, just have them jerk you off or get head, or masturbate them. I think masturbation is wonderful because it keeps a lot of diseases out of the equation usually and it definitely won't let anyone get pregnant.

CHIP Z'NUFF: If you don't have anything at all, just don't come inside them and when the act is finished make sure she gets up and goes to the bathroom and pees. Then the guy should go to the bathroom and wash up and clean up, for sure. That's the best thing you can do. You're taking a chance. If it's with somebody you don't know really well that's the way the game is played. One in every four kids has STDs right now, but in our generation I'm not so sure it was like that. In the old days when you'd catch something you'd take something and you were OK in seven days to go out fucking again. Nowadays it's a lot tougher.

COURTNEY TAYLOR-TAYLOR: Mutual masturbation.

DANKO JONES: Just walk away and jerk off. I would do that, just jerk off. I couldn't be bothered because the next week-and-a-half you're going to be a zombie scared out of your mind with who or what you spent the night with.

DOUG ROBB: I guess it depends who you're hooking up with. If it's someone that you've been in a relationship with for a while and you know their history and know they don't have any STDs or anything, and you don't feel totally worried about pregnancy, you could give it a shot anyway because it feels better. But if it's somebody you don't know, I would just say don't do it, geez.

GINGER: Do not fuck! Practise your foreplay skills and bring her to a long and satisfying climax with oral sex. Plenty of hugs afterwards too. You will definitely get to use those new condoms you're going to buy tomorrow.

HANDSOME DICK MANITOBA: Me, if I was doing it and knew we were fooling around, I would say, 'I don't have any, you don't have any, I don't know your history, you don't know my history, let's have some fun and we'll do more next time.' Something like that. 'Let's have some fun and play with each other.' There's lots of fun to be had without catching diseases.

JAMES KOTTAK: Split!

JIMMY ASHHURST: If you don't have any condoms it's like, 'Sorry mate, you're going to be handling it yourself.' Jerking off is good and she gets to stick around for it if she's keen. That's as far as it's going to go though... maybe a little oral.

LEMMY: Do it without one, I suppose. I can't use one anyway; I can't do it. I just crack up laughing. The only time I ever tried to use one I fell off the bed laughing, and she was laughing as well. So she didn't get pregnant, because you can't get pregnant from laughing.

NICKE BORG: Don't have sex; don't penetrate – don't do that.

ROB PATTERSON: Nothing, don't do it.

TOBY RAND: A whole lot of foreplay… or wing it. Just pray!

VAZQUEZ: You just can't do it man – get a blowjob instead.

Once in a relationship, how do you decide whether it's the pill or condoms?

ACEY SLADE: It's a place where I'm kind of old-fashioned in a way. With my ex before my wife, we used condoms the whole time we were together; never once didn't use a condom because we weren't engaged and we weren't married, so we used them the whole time. Because we weren't engaged, it wasn't a monogamous relationship, so there was no way I was going to put her at risk. But with my wife, once we were engaged, then I stopped using a condom. So for me, it's about where it's going to end up going, because God forbid you have sex with someone and you knock them up and you end up having a kid in this world and that wasn't the intention. I will only have sex without a condom if I think I have a future with the person.

ADDE: The thing about Swedish girls is that *every* Swedish girl is on a pill – it's a promiscuous country. But really, as soon as you start a relationship with somebody, you lose the condom.

ALLISON ROBERTSON: I guess that depends on the person. Some girls want to take pills and some don't. Some girls can't either because it affects them or something, so you might always have to use a condom. I think it completely depends. I think girls should take the pill if they want. I think that's good. Even if you don't have sex, it's just a good thing. Usually they help protect against cancer and stuff, so I think the pill is a nice thing. If you want to get pregnant, then it's not.

BLASKO: I think it's up to the girl. Some girls don't like to be on the pill. If they're smokers they really can't be on the pill. So I think the ball's in their court generally.

BRENT MUSCAT: I've done both. I had a girlfriend and we used the condom as a form of protection for like three years and then I've had girlfriends who used the pill and we didn't use condoms. So I guess the main thing is if you're not going to use condoms, you want to know that hopefully they're not sleeping with anyone else.

DANKO JONES: It's not for me to decide. It's more her because it's her body.

JESSE HUGHES: No glove, no love. I'm a bareback rider myself; I'm a cowboy baby!

JIMMY ASHHURST: Oh God, if you're in a relationship then fuck the condoms off. Enough is enough.

NICKE BORG: There's so much stuff about pills making girls go emotionally fucking disturbed and where girls changed pills and nothing fucking changes, yet some did stop and they turned out to be a totally different person. So I don't know; that's really weird. I don't like pills in general, whether it's for you having a mental disease or you don't want to get pregnant; I don't like pills to fuck with your body because they *are* fucking with you. And also it would be really boring to have to use a condom all the time, so I guess… There is something called a Persona. It's like a little fertility machine and it tells you exactly when your partner can come in you or he has to pull it out before. It is actually very, very specific – not in hours, but absolutely days. It looks like a little cell phone actually. You can look at it and see, 'Go ahead, fill me up, but tomorrow you have to wait for three days.' It's awesome!

TOBY RAND: I think there's a way to do it without either of them. I'm a big fan of if the girl doesn't want to take the pill – fine. I won't wear a condom, so long as we've both been checked and we're all cool, and then any time before I'm about to come we find other ways to get me off without being inside her. I love that. I love coming on the exterior, rather than being inside. I love it.

VAZQUEZ: Definitely the pill because let's face it, I fucking hate condoms. They're a necessary evil, but condoms are for guys with short hair!

What's the best way to be safe when moving from one orifice to another?

ACEY SLADE: Showers, condoms.

BLASKO: I've heard that's a big no-no. I've heard you're not really meant to be doing that.

DANKO JONES: If you want to do it the proper way, sometimes it can definitely kill the mood when you have to scoot off and clean off. I don't know man.

ROB PATTERSON: That makes me laugh!

TOBY RAND: If there's a bathroom handy, there's nothing better than to go and jump in the shower for a quick rinse. Once I had some juice beside the bed – I think it was a vodka and orange – and I just grabbed it out and washed my dick. You know, girls are pretty good like that. They look after themselves.

ONCE I HAD SOME JUICE BESIDE THE BED – I THINK IT WAS A VODKA AND ORANGE – AND I JUST GRABBED IT OUT AND WASHED MY DICK.

VAZQUEZ: This is important: if you're going from her pussy to her ass, it's like you cannot go back in her pussy after. If you're really doing a lot of fucking anal, you've got to make sure you shower after and I'll tell you why: it's not really for the guy, it's for the girl. You get like urinary tract infections and they're like, 'I really want you to fuck me in the ass' and you're like, 'Oh great!' You definitely want to do the clean up after.

SEXUAL PREFERENCE
(HETERO & HOMO)

"THE WAY TO TELL IF YOUR BEST FRIEND IS GAY IS TO SEE IF HIS DICK TASTES LIKE SHIT"

How do you know if you have gay or bisexual tendencies?

ACEY SLADE: Oh, 'All rock'n'roll is homesexual.' That's a quote from someone in a band like the Manic Street Preachers. I don't know. I don't feel like I've ever had any tendencies.

ADDE: If you get attracted to a man that's when you get at least bisexual.

ALLISON ROBERTSON: I grew up so liberal in California, I think that everybody could be a little bit gay if they wanted to and it's only a matter of unlocking that part of the brain or not. I don't think there's anything wrong with maybe thinking you might be and choosing not to be; it's completely up to the person. I feel maybe you should go out of the closet if you just know that you're pretty much interested in one sex. If you're confused, I think there's nothing wrong with keeping it to yourself until you're ready. To me, I feel like you just know. I think people know; I think a lot of people know from the second they are born and it takes a long time to feel comfortable sometimes.

ANDREW W.K.: That's a very perplexing question that I'm sure people have wondered about for their whole lives. When is someone gay, when is someone bi? Is it because of ideas they've had, things they've done? Can you have done something and still say you're straight? Can you have desires and never follow them and still say that you're gay or straight? I mean, these are very esoteric questions. Some people would say you're born gay and to deny it is like to deny you're a certain race. Other people say to label yourself any way, including a sexuality, is a confusion based on your ability to make free choice at every moment. So I guess each person figures out the way that they feel comfortable with looking at their sexuality and then they work from that. I've heard stories of friends of mine who I think are straight men but they've had experiences where… to me, even having sexual experiences where there's another man present, whether you end up doing anything with them, that to me is pretty intense. But I've had straight friends that think of that as a very straight activity. You're looking at different levels of what it is to be gay. There are some people that think so long as you don't get fucked – another man can give you a blowjob or you can fuck another man – that's not being gay. These ideas are clearly very personal and very broad and it really only comes down to the individual. I think the main thing is to just not be concerned so much with what you are but to follow more what you want to do and I guess that's just been really challenging for society to look at in that way. I've never had a gay experience and it's not something that has occurred to me, but I would even give myself the freedom to say that sexuality is a very vast place and I don't want to limit anybody, including myself ultimately.

BRENT MUSCAT: Well if you're attracted to someone of the same sex, I guess you'd be at least bi. If you're a guy and you're not attracted to girls and you look at guys and think, 'Wow! He's sexy' and you don't think girls are sexy, then I guess you would know that you are gay. I think it would be pretty obvious.

BRUCE KULICK: Obviously, if you're attracted to guys you're gay. Not saying there's anything wrong with that. I think guys usually know it at a fairly young age. It's not like suddenly at 40 you become gay; you usually know it in high school. I can recognise a handsome guy and say, 'Wow that guy is handsome.' I know when an actor is a good-looking guy, or a musician is. When I grew up and I saw The Beatles, I knew McCartney was a really attractive guy; all the guys in The Beatles were good-looking in their own way. It's easy to say someone's attractive, but then if you're gay you're imagining kissing them and sleeping with them. I don't think it's that complicated really. I've always had a thing for women, yet I like clothes and I like fashion and presenting myself (for the most part) neatly. Sometimes I'll use the term 'I'm metrosexual', but there's a big difference between metrosexual and gay of course.

CHIP Z'NUFF: Well you'd know right away, because if you're a guy and you're attracted to another guy, you're bisexual. If you want to kiss a guy… I think men are attractive OK, but I don't want to fuck them. I can see a guy who's good-looking and I can say to my chick, 'You know what? He's a really handsome cat.' Like if you're walking down the street and you're holding hands and she goes, 'Wow, that guy's good-looking.' I can go, 'Yeah he is. He's very handsome.' But if you look at that guy and you want to kiss him, you're bisexual. It's not anything to be ashamed of if you are, it's just that's what it is. I grew up in a family of boys and girls and I'm pretty cool about that stuff. I've seen both sides of it. I know I love my chicks.

COURTNEY TAYLOR-TAYLOR: I don't know. I've never really felt like I had, but here's what Brian Warner said: 'If you're sucking another guy's dick and you have a hard-on, you're gay. If you don't have a hard-on, you're not.' That was Marilyn Manson's take on that, which I always think is funny, so I'll just say that's how.

DANKO JONES: I guess you just want to have sex with the same sex. I'm pretty straight. I'm around dudes all the time and never has that thought entered my head. I guess once you have that thought, you pretty much sign up for those types of sexuality.

DOUG ROBB: The same way you would know if you have straight tendencies. It's not like you decide, 'Hmm, I like vagina.' I know I have straight tendencies. If you start to go, 'I like vagina, but then again I like dick sometimes', then you'd be telling yourself, 'I'm bi.' I think you just know.

HANDSOME DICK MANITOBA: I like what the comedian Andrew Dice Clay said: 'What's with this bisexuality? There's no such thing as bisexuality. You either suck cock or you don't!' That was his attitude and it always rang true with me.

JESSE HUGHES: The best way to know if you're gay is if you have a giant erection while giving your best friend a blowjob. The way to tell if your best friend is gay is to see if his dick tastes like shit.

JIMMY ASHHURST: If you find yourself with a dick up your ass then the chances are you're gay.

LEMMY: Probably when your boyfriend's cock tastes of shit.

NICKE BORG: There is this old school thing (which I feel sorry for everyone that reads this; I'm going to get slapped by a bunch of chicks for this): most girls have this urge to have sex with another female. Most guys don't have that thing to have sex with another guy. I don't really get turned on by, 'Do you want me to lick my sister or best friend?' I'm like, 'Well fine, yeah, if she wants to.' But it would be really, really horrible to get dumped because of a girl. That would make you feel really stupid, and I've seen a lot of similar things where men get dumped by their wife or whatever for another girl… or the other way around. 'I'm sorry we have two kids but I'm gay and I'm going to marry Mr Paul right now.' It'd be like, 'What the fuck?' That must be really hard for somebody to take that. 'I've been with you for 10 years and we'd fuck, and now you're gay?' I have a lot of gay friends, including guys, and I love them all.

ROB PATTERSON: Suck a dick. If you like it, you'll know.

TOBY RAND: I know that I don't because I know that I can appreciate a good-looking guy but I definitely don't want to make out with them. But then again, I'm very affectionate with my guy friends.

VAZQUEZ: I think you're just born that way. I think it's just one of those things. I'm a total believer in you're either born gay or you're not – and that's that. I mean, I love women's clothes, but…

What's your preferred reply to someone of the same sex hitting on you?

ACEY SLADE: I think it's flattering but it's just, 'Hey man, I don't swing that way.' Just like Led Zeppelin – there is no *In Through The Out Door*.

ADDE: I'll be nice but really, really... like a gentleman but really cold, you know.

ALLISON ROBERTSON: I guess I just don't want to be mean or them to think I'm offended, because I'm never offended by that, so I usually just say, 'That's really sweet of you but I don't like girls like that.' It's a compliment, so I never want to say something that would be like, 'Eeww.' I actually think it's nicer sometimes to be hit on by a girl than some weird dude. It's more of a compliment sometimes or seems gentler. Not always though!

ANDREW W.K.: It's actually not happened to me very frequently and I've been very grateful for that, because the times it has have been very awkward. I've just had to say, 'I'm sorry. I'm not interested. I'm not into that' or 'I have a girlfriend' or 'I'm married' or 'I'm straight.' It's just weird. It's just been weird. It's not something that I would ever hope to have happen again. But it's also very similar to when a woman does it and you're just not interested in that woman; it's been equally uncomfortable to do that. There were times when I had to say that to a woman and it was just painful to say I'm not interested in being with you; it's just harsh.

BLASKO: 'Dude, I don't swing that way.'

BRENT MUSCAT: I've had a lot of guys doing that in the past, a lot of guys hitting on me. I usually don't say anything. So long as they're not trying to touch me or make me feel uncomfortable. I guess I would say that I have a girlfriend. I wouldn't want to insult anyone. I would just say I have a girlfriend and they'd figure I'm straight.

BRUCE KULICK: I had an apartment in a very hip area of L.A. in West Hollywood so it would occasionally happen, but no one has obviously hit on me. I had one neighbour who was a little flirty in that way, but I wasn't going to go there; that's ridiculous. I don't know that gay guys generally put out that energy on us; they kind of know if they're going to have a shot. I think that's why I haven't run into it much.

CHIP Z'NUFF: 'Oh thank you very much. I really appreciate it. I'm totally flattered that you think I'm attractive, but I've got a girlfriend and she trips my trigger. I'm sure you're going to find what you're looking for because you're very easy on the eyes.' Make them feel good. Don't be disrespectful to them. It's flattering for anybody to think you're attractive. A negative response like, 'Get the fuck away from me!' only makes it look like you might be gay or bisexual and you're just afraid to embrace your feelings.

COURTNEY TAYLOR-TAYLOR: I think I usually just say something like, 'Dude, not so much with the faggotry.'

DANKO JONES: Oh I'm totally cool with that; that's happened before. I don't take it as an insult. I actually take it as a compliment. I just go, 'I'm straight. Sorry man. I like girls.' And then they go, 'You think you like girls' and that whole thing. No, that's great. It's cool by me. I don't care. It's a compliment, definitely.

DOUG ROBB: At this moment, I just kind of hold my hand up and show the [wedding] ring.

HANDSOME DICK MANITOBA: That rarely happens. I'm just not a cute type. I don't think I get the classic homosexual come-on. You have to be more of a pretty boy or something, I don't know. It rarely happens that somebody is coming onto to me where I have to say something. I've heard people say, 'Everyone is gay, everyone is bisexual, it's just that they don't get around to it' or something like that. Whatever, I don't know. Maybe it's true, maybe it's not. Maybe I'll find out one day, maybe I won't. Right now, I'm completely enamoured with vaginas, tits and kissing, and I've never really needed to swing on chandeliers with 19 people to give me an erection.

JAMES KOTTAK: 'Thanks dude, you'd make an excellent wife.'

JESSE HUGHES: 'As long as we don't kiss, anything goes, because I ain't no queer.'

JIMMY ASHHURST: 'Well, thank you very much.'

LEMMY: 'Thanks but no thanks,' basically.

NICKE BORG: My reply would be, 'Dude, I'm very flattered. I think you're great; I think you're fucking cool. Dude, we can hang – but do not fucking touch me. I'm not going to be gay because we fucking drink or do drugs.' Usually gay people are very open and easier to talk to about stuff in general. So I'd be like, 'Dude, I'm very flattered, thank you very much, but I'm not. Even if you drug me with the best fucking blow and get me whatever – sorry!'

ROB PATTERSON: 'I'm straight, dude. Sorry. I'm flattered though, thank you.'

TOBY RAND: My preferred reply is to say, 'Nah mate. You're awesome. Let's just hang and have some fun' because I've met a lot of gay guys and they've never been really, really forward – they've shown interest. I think the best way is to laugh and kind of have fun with it and just chill out with them; make them feel cool. Just like anyone; if you're letting someone down you can still hang out with them and be friends – who cares?

VAZQUEZ: Oh man, I think it's hysterical. I'm very gracious about that. 'It's cool, man. I know I'm gorgeous.' If a guy wants to tell me I'm gorgeous, I'm like, 'Hey man, thanks.'

What's the best way to set up a threesome, or moresome?

ACEY SLADE: Unfortunately there's usually booze involved with that. I think generally, just getting two girls in a room alone with you with a bottle of Jack Daniel's – if either of those girls can't figure out what's going to happen, then they're pretty dumb.

ADDE: I think it has to be like… if I want to have a threesome, it has to be with strangers. It's not something you do with friends at all.

ALLISON ROBERTSON: I've never done that but I would have to say that no matter who you are or which part of the three you are, you have to be ready for it to be a disaster, or not. You have to be prepared for it to go awry or for it to end up in not the way you thought it would be. So I say the best way to set it up is to be careful going about it and make sure you really feel comfortable. I would also say just be prepared that you might not see the other two ever again.

ANDREW W.K.: Wow! I've never done that either and whether it's two women or two men, that's just very intense. It involves a third consciousness. The closest I've got to that even in the most remote way is watching pornography while being with a woman. Even though you're watching it on video, it's a third perspective, a third point of view, it's something else to engage in and look at. You can do that similar to if you picture someone else in your head or have a fantasy going while you're having sex, but to actually have a third person there is just really over the top. I would look forward to that experience in theory, but it's something where you're unleashing an energy that's extremely powerful and possibly destructive and is risky. It seems just very, very intense.

BLASKO: I think it's hard to convince one person to bring on another. It kind of has to organically be there already. Like, you kind of have to be in a situation where girls are teeing it up in the first place.

BRENT MUSCAT: In the past when it's happened to me, it's usually been the girls that have approached me or kind of said, 'Hey, me and my friend want to do it', but maybe because I was in the band I was lucky. If the girl you're with is into girls, I guess you could always say, 'Hey what about that girl, what about this girl?' I guess you just keep trying until you find the one. If you've got one who's ready to go, then it's just a numbers game. Some guys are so brave they'd ask

1,000 girls and get turned down 999 times, but there's just that one time and that's all you need.

BRUCE KULICK: If you're in a relationship, you've obviously got to think, 'Would that person be willing to do that?' I think there are less girls that want another girl… firstly, a guy usually doesn't want another guy in the picture; you want another girl. If my current girlfriend was willing to do that, I would still be really nervous about doing it because I just think it opens up a lot of questions in general that might in some ways make a problem in the relationship. So I keep it more in that fantasy category. If it has happened for somebody in a good way then great, good for them, but I just don't think it's that easy.

CHIP Z'NUFF: The first thing to do is talk. Talk to your partner about a threesome. If you're by yourself and you're going to be with two girls – a man meets two girls – just invite them both over to your pad and hang out a little. Have some glasses of wine there maybe, a couple of joints to smoke a little bit and just chat and converse. If you feel that that could happen before you even get there, then it's pretty much a no-brainer. Let the girls start first though. That's what I recommend. You sit back and stay out of the way. Don't be this smothering jag-off. Then once the girls start going, then you can judge and decide what your next move is going to be. But let them start it first. That's my recommendation and I know that works.

COURTNEY TAYLOR-TAYLOR: I think they're a bad idea; someone's feelings are going to get hurt.

DANKO JONES: Find a girl who's into that shit because there's no sense in forcing a girl who's not into that to try it. It's obvious that it could ruin the relationship. It's not worth it. Well, it depends: if you don't care about the relationship, then by all means force the issue, but if you care about the relationship forcing the issue might ruin the relationship. It's just best to find someone pre-packaged for that with those tendencies already.

DOUG ROBB: How do you set that type of magic up? I think it just goes back to being open about it; throw it out there and say this is something you're into. If your partner's into it, maybe it'll happen some time. If your partner says they're not into it, it ain't going to happen.

GINGER: Have her choose the girl. And you will want her to do this again, so make sure to spend a lot more time and eye contact on your woman, no matter how much you want to devour her friend.

HANDSOME DICK MANITOBA: Did you ever see the TV show *Curb Your Enthusiasm*? It's a great comedy show here on HBO and one time for their 10-year anniversary the wife said, 'You can have another girl, one day on your 10th year,' so I bring that up as a joke to my wife sometimes. We've thought about it. She's actually said, 'If that's something you really want to do, we can do it' and I thought about it and just thought it could be really fun, but it could also have long-lasting implications. Like, if I like the girl too much, or if she gets really jealous I'm touching the girl on whatever body part or kissing the girl, or there's any sort of intimacy, or what if *they* hit it off and that bothers me? There's one thing that can go right: you enjoy it in the moment, you have fun for the day and you let it go. But if by some chance you have a hard time letting it go, you're going to have lingering memories. Either your wife is going to have lingering memories of you being too involved, or you might. There's a bunch of things that could go wrong. Every once in a while I think about it. I think one day we're going to do it. I think what we would do is set up a situation – because I'd like to do it – but I think we'd set up a situation where it's pretty guaranteed that it's just going to be light fun. But you never know, I don't know. We talk about it and we haven't got around to it yet, but I think one day we might.

JESSE HUGHES: Do it with math teachers.

JIMMY ASHHURST: Oh that's touchy shit man! Some of the weirdest shit has resulted from that. Like, the weirdest emotional shit, even if they're game at first. You'd better make damn sure that they're both game first, especially if one of them is one that you care about. Chances are that it's all going to be fun and games in the beginning, but then you're in for it once the other one leaves! I think the best way is if they're both acquaintances. Once you're in a relationship I'm afraid, unless you're way more skilled than I, then it's best to stay away from that.

LEMMY: Usually it's the girl that suggests it actually, in a successful one. Guys suggesting it usually don't go down that well because chicks feel insulted and shit all the time. It's very easy to put the thing the wrong way, especially if you're not very good with words.

NICKE BORG: I think it's not really up to you, it's up to the female. For me as a guy, it must be an idea coming from your girlfriend or wife or whatever. And then, you should just be like, 'I don't know; I'm not sure. Are you sure baby?' 'Yeah, I want to do it.' Then you're like, 'OK baby' and then it's, 'Fuck yeah!'

TOBY RAND: The best way to do it is to kiss a girl and then also show interest in her friend. Actually, I think the best way to do it is to find the right girls because until then… they're out there. Actually last weekend I experienced it – true story. I was at the pub and this one girl goes… I was going to go to a house party and she goes, 'No, I want you to stay' and I'm like, 'I don't know if I should' and she goes, 'All right' so she made out with me. So I looked at her friend standing nearby and I said, 'I think I might go,' so she said to her friend, 'Come over here – you can make out with him as well.' So I made out with her, then we all made out – so I stayed.

VAZQUEZ: That's happened to me very rarely but it always happened when I least expected it. With an ex-girlfriend of mine, it was just weird: we were having all these problems in our relationship and it looked like we were ready to break up. She was staying at my house and her best friend was staying at my house as well. The three of us were on the couch and all this tension's going on because the relationship's ending. Then the next thing you know, the three of us are just going at it. Dude, it was weird because most girls don't want to do that with their best friend. It was probably one of the weirdest experiences of my life as I didn't see that coming at all!

When is it OK for others on the outside to know of your sexual preferences?

JESSE HUGHES: Honestly, from the time I was a little kid, my Mum worked in a department store called Bullets and she had a lot of gay friends. Gay people are some of the most fun people in the world, truly. Where I grew up in the South, interestingly enough, to be gay in the South you have to be fucking tough. Like, just consider this: the first rock'n'roller was a gay, black dude from the South named Little Richard. I can't imagine a tougher spot to be in, ever!
To do that, you end up being like Fred Schneider from the B-52s, weird and tough as shit. When I moved to San Francisco, I learned something really quick: gay dudes can fuck you up! They can fight like sons of bitches and they can come out swinging. Then I learned that there are two types of homosexuals: there's trauma gay and Roman or Greek gay. Trauma gay is where something bad happened to you as a child that made you focus on yourself and fixate upon your own sexual identity for whatever reason and you end up being a drag queen or having a sex alteration or whatever. Then there's Roman gays, the ones that I believe were born gay. Those are the ones that look at themselves and go, 'Oh my God, this is hot! I want to do it with this', and they just date someone that looks exactly like them ie body builders and actors. A lot of the gay community loves to be men. When you go around San Francisco and you see the Bear and Cuffs shit – holy God! You can't help but see from my style that there's something I love about the gay community.

ROB PATTERSON: I don't care either way. I'm an open book.

TECHNIQUE IMPROVEMENTS

"IF YOU MAKE A GIRL SQUIRT YOU FEEL LIKE A FUCKING GOD; IT'S FUCKING FANTASTIC"

What do you find drives them crazy every time?

ACEY SLADE: Stamina, going the distance.

TOBY RAND: I love talking in the ear. I like to grab the back of their hair really hard and bite their neck. It all depends on the mood of the sex as well, because if it's passionate, hard sex like that, then definitely pulling the hair and using mirrors and telling them, 'Watch this' and guiding them through it – that's always a lot of fun.

VAZQUEZ: You've just got to last, man. That's it – you cannot come in two minutes. The only time I'm going to come in two minutes is if I'm doing it on purpose because I just don't give a fuck. 'I've already performed tonight, I'm done.' Really though, you have to be able to last; you have to. Let's face it: women never get fucked the right way.

How can new techniques be learnt?

ACEY SLADE: I feel like I learn more from my partners telling me what they like; so paying attention.

ADDE: From meeting a lot of girls and really being interested in what's happening.

BLASKO: I think there's never anything wrong with asking questions. I think there's never anything wrong with experimenting. Being shy isn't really all that sexy. It's like, 'Hey can I try this?' or, 'Let's do this.' So, asking questions and then trying different things – I think anyone would be open to that.

DANKO JONES: Just by never getting into a rut in bed by doing the same strokes every single time. If you vary it up a bit, eventually you'll stumble on something that's actually new and exciting for the both of you. That's how I find it. You just don't do the same strokes every single time you jump into bed. There's got to be something that's different. And I notice as soon as I'm getting into a rut, it just gets boring and I want to change it up anyway.

JIMMY ASHHURST: It's like life; it's a work in progress. Practice makes perfect. If at first you don't succeed, try, try again.

TOBY RAND: I think watching porn; it's always good fun. I think it's also about just breaking down your inhibitions and just trying shit you've always wanted. I think using a mirror – definitely – because you can see the way their body moves. You can tell by their actions if they're enjoying it or not.

VAZQUEZ: Definitely through porn.

What's the best way to test-drive a new technique?

JIMMY ASHHURST: With someone you're comfortable with hopefully. If you can find that one who's game for anything, then you put her in the back of the phone book for sure.

ROB PATTERSON: Try it!

VAZQUEZ: I love fucking girls in the ass. A lot of girls are really apprehensive because like some guy tried to do it to them when they were like 16 and fucking did it all wrong and shit and they were hurt. So my advice for that, if you're going to fuck a girl in the ass for the first time, you're going to have to warm them up to it. You're going to have to use the fingers, then you work up to the small dildo in the ass. Then when you're going to do it to them, the best way to start is when they're on their back and lift their legs back. Usually in porn you see them bent over, but that's the pro's position – that's when a girl's ass can handle anything. At first, the best thing you can do is have them lying on the bed, preferably on the corner so you can stand on the floor, take it in slow and you're all set. Dude, women fucking love it man. It's crazy.

Know any slight intercourse improvements to really heighten sexual response?

ROB PATTERSON: Be passionate. Passion, passion, passion. It's all about emotions!

VAZQUEZ: If you can make a woman feel really comfortable with herself, her whole experience is going to be that much better. If they feel sexy and they don't feel weird at all, they go fucking bananas, man. One time in my life I was with a girl who squirts and I was so excited man. At that point, I'd only seen it in porn and I had no idea. Dude, it was fucking awesome, because when you make a girl come you feel like the hero but if she fucking squirts, your ego goes through the fucking roof! If you make a girl squirt, you feel like a fucking God; it's fucking fantastic.

TOYS & TOOLS

"I GOT A COCK RING A WHILE BACK AND IT ACTUALLY WORKS. IT HEIGHTENS THE PLEASURE. IT'S LIKE I CAN'T REALLY LIVE WITHOUT IT ANYMORE"

What's the strangest sex toy you've seen?

ACEY SLADE: I saw a girl get fucked by another girl's foot; that was pretty weird.

ALLISON ROBERTSON: We used to go over to Big Al's in San Francisco. It's like a really big warehouse of sex toys and stuff. I've never cared about that stuff personally, as far as needing it. I think it's fun to look at it and play around and see what's there. I always thought (I know they're not that weird any more) that the blow-up dolls are just kind of weird. I don't care how normal other people think they are, they always make me feel like, 'Woah! That's just so silly.' Like, I don't know how anybody could have them around and not think they're funny, but I know that some people really do use them. To me that's more comical than sexy.

ANDREW W.K.: When I was in Amsterdam for the first time, I was 13. My Dad and I went on a European trip and Amsterdam was one of the places we visited for two or three days and I had never been exposed to that much sexuality in any period of my life up to that point. It was just completely over the top walking down the street and going past store windows that had every possible type of vibrator, sex toy and pornography playing on video. It was just a very transformative time in my life and I still think about it all the time; it was that powerful. It was one of my first sexual experiences where I was seeing other people have sex like that. I'd seen porn before but never like this. There were some toys there that I'm not sure that I still understand what they did; those with three parts on them to stimulate all three main areas on a woman but each protrusion was shaped like a different animal and sculptured in almost a cartoonish level of realism. That to me was pretty disturbing but really amazing too, just to think that some artist had first drawn this out, that a group of people (mostly men I imagined) had sat around and said, 'OK, here's what we're going to make. We work in this company that makes these kinds of sex toys and here's the new one we're going to design' and some guy had to sculpt that. Then most likely they tested it and then it was available and people go buy it and take it home. That was just over the top.

BLASKO: Something I thought was fucking hilarious: it was probably intentionally made for lesbians and it's like a chin strap and on the chin is a dildo, so that would be going in the pussy while whoever is licking the clit, and it was called The Accommodator! I think that is fucking hilarious.

BRENT MUSCAT: We played an adult film museum the other night. There's a guy from England who's a hydraulics specialist and he made all kinds of strange contraptions. He made a race car where you would sit down – almost like a bobsled – and you face forward and the girl sits in it and drives it around a race track. There was a dildo that would go in and out of her as she was driving and the faster she would go, the faster the dildo would go. He made like three of these little race cars and he had some kind of race with these different girls doing it. He had all kinds of weird stuff where the girl would be getting screwed in the butt with one; it was like a machine. It was a little scary; it was frightening. It looked like something out of the movie *Saw*. That's probably the strangest contraption I've seen.

BRUCE KULICK: They certainly sell some vibrators that look insane, but I always go back to the *Austin Powers* thing – the thing that supposedly makes your penis larger or something. That's so silly in that movie and I'm glad he goofed on it because it's kind of silly. There are some really intense vibrators that supposedly some women love, but I haven't dated a lot of girls who were into the whole vibrator thing, even though that would be fun for me. I wouldn't have a problem playing with one and bringing a toy into it, but I've got to admit, most of my girls have been more organic about everything and that's fine with me.

CHIP Z'NUFF: There was a dildo with three different pieces on it, coming out from three different sides. So if there are other people there, more than one person can participate. It had a little button on there and it would make this motorised noise and it would turn in circles like you're circle-pumping somebody. That was pretty interesting.

COURTNEY TAYLOR-TAYLOR: I don't know; I don't really live in that world much.

DANKO JONES: A 10-inch dildo that stuck to the wall! The sex store that I worked at in like '99 was mainly porno and they had a wall of sex toys and stuff. Blow-up dolls were always weird; when guys came in for blow-up dolls, that was always really weird. I just always thought that blow-up dolls were the weirdest fucking things. I mean, when they didn't snicker like it was supposed to be a party gag and they got their friends to buy it because their buddy's getting married or something – a gag like that is one thing, but those aren't the people I sold them to. They were like some serious dudes who really wanted to make sure that the lips were fine and the vagina was nice and tight. It was just really weird! It was just a weird sell. I just couldn't believe I was having a serious conversation with someone about a blow-up doll and how well it worked. Blow-up dolls are just used as gags and props for most people you know, but the people that came into the store were pretty weird.

DOUG ROBB: I've only had experience with a couple, but I've seen some strange shit on TV that's for sure. A couple of the guys in my band got me this fake vagina years ago for my birthday. It had two holes and the whole deal.

It looked like a real-sized vagina and inside it had all these weird rubber fingers or something like that, and it broke after two times. That is not a statement about me packing any type of heat or anything! It was just a piece of shit; it didn't even feel like it.

EVAN SEINFELD: It's got to be a toss-up between something called the RealDoll – it's a life-like, like $6,000 doll that actually looks so much like a real woman it's kind of creepy. It's like fucking a dead person or an android or something. So a toss-up between that and then down in San Francisco there's a couple of like gay leather shops, and I'm a big fan of quality leather, but they happen to stock a few items like a rubber arm and fist and I've even seen this rubber kind of fire hydrant thing.

HANDSOME DICK MANITOBA: I used to date a girl in the Seventies who answered phones. There's always been a big connection between dancers and prostitutes and rock'n'roll, and I dated a girl that worked at the most famous S&M house in New York that was called Belle de Jour. They had this room that was full of devices for torture and they would tell me that some men would let themselves be humiliated or hung upside down, or put diapers on. They had to be spanked or humiliated to get an erection, so that whole world… Like, I actually went to some of those parties and it was so out there to me, that whole world. I've seen stuff, I'm aware of stuff, but I haven't used it in my personal life.

I JUST COULDN'T BELIEVE I WAS HAVING A SERIOUS CONVERSATION WITH SOMEONE ABOUT A BLOW-UP DOLL AND HOW WELL IT WORKED.

JAMES KOTTAK: We were in Germany and we thought there was a camera or something in the roof and we found this huge, big ball thing. We don't know what it was to this day. I've never seen anything like it. It looked like a plumbing device.

JESSE HUGHES: A party sheep – an inflatable sheep.

JIMMY ASHHURST: They're doing pretty good with latex these days, doing amazing things. And those crazy life-like fucking dolls they have now where they're borderline human – RealDolls. A friend of mine had one of those fucking things; that's some crazy shit. The most freaky thing I've ever seen. He didn't share her.

LEMMY: I think Ben Wa Balls are really weird. Our guitar player once asked a runner going out for some food to get some Chinese food and an extra portion of

Ben Wa Balls. The guy ran out and he came back and he got them. He obviously went to a sex shop and bought a set. Fucking excellent – a good guy; he called his bluff. I think it was in Australia actually.

NICKE BORG: Dude, these days people are just fucking nuts, man. I went to this fucking old castle in southern France, like a museum and an old vineyard. In the corner was this little setup with dildos. I'm in a centuries-old castle and here they are selling dildos – so everything has changed. I'm kind of immune. Sex toys are fun in a way but I've never really been that… If I was a girl and couldn't possibly find a partner, I'd go look and would probably be overloaded with fucking toys. So the weirdest one? I wouldn't know. I had a double-dong dildo once.

ROB PATTERSON: A tube that shoots milk into an ass.

TOBY RAND: It was like a shoehorn; it seriously was! I was like, 'What does that do?' The girl actually put it in… it was a really long spoon-looking kind of thing, and she put it in and was almost like scooping herself with it. And then I put my dick on it and it would slide in as well, and while my dick was in there I could feel the end of the spoon on the top of my dick. It was really weird and I was wondering what it was doing for her but I guess it kind of felt like the head of my dick was the spoon as well for her. She could twist it over; it was really interesting – really cool.

VAZQUEZ: Jesus man, you go to a store anywhere around here and you'll see all kinds of fucked-up shit. Nothing stands out though, it's all pretty normal. In my fucked-up head it's all normal.

What's the best toy for taking them right over the top?

ACEY SLADE: The rabbit. That's the one that has the part that comes over the top that tickles the clit and has a vibrator. That seems to work pretty good.

ADDE: The cock ring! I got a cock ring a while back and it actually works. It heightens the pleasure. It's like I can't really live without it any more.

ALLISON ROBERTSON: I never had to use any really, but I've heard people talking about the cock ring you put on with the little vibrator thing on it. I've heard people rave about that. I don't know. I've never really had to use anything. I'm lucky like that I guess.

BLASKO: Everybody's different. You kind of have to experiment, so I don't think there's one thing that works for everybody.

BRENT MUSCAT: I'm 41 now and sometimes I think there's already a generation gap, where young girls now talk about, 'Oh I have a vibrator' and they'll talk about which ones they like. When I was growing up, I never heard girls talk about that. If any of my girlfriends had them they would keep it secret, but girls nowadays are very open about it. I've heard the Pocket Rocket is the one the girls go crazy for.

SO IF YOU USE ONE OF THOSE SMALL DILDOS UP THEIR ASS WHILE YOU'RE FUCKING THEM AT THE SAME TIME, THEY GO BANANAS!

CHIP Z'NUFF: From what I hear those little butterflies are really good. You just put it around the clitoris and hold it on there. You can kiss them down that way while they've got that on there and they can have multiple orgasms if used the right way. Don't press it too hard.

DOUG ROBB: My guitar player gave me this thing that was almost like a jelly, latex cock ring. It looks like a collar that a St Bernard wears with the little wooden barrel, but the wooden barrel is a tiny vibrator or something like that. [Ed: He asks his guitarist about it.] He says he thinks they call them o-rings. But if you put it upside down so the little thing is on top, when you're having sex that's vibrating the girl's clit. I don't know if it took her over the top but it was pretty fucking funny to put on and try and explain.

JAMES KOTTAK: I've heard it's a vibrator but I wouldn't be one to know. Natural is always the best.

JESSE HUGHES: The one called my genitals… Nah, I'm just joking. Actually the Pocket Rocket is the one I've heard most requested.

JIMMY ASHHURST: The rabbit: it's a dildo with the little extra bit that vibrates. It's good stuff. There's this other one that you stick in and it's got a remote control on it so you can be at the other end of the bar or out some place and give her a little zap – that's awesome! It makes for a fun night out man, especially if she's got a sense of humour. You can wait until she's engaged in a very serious conversation and then buzz and give her a fucking jolt. That's always good.

LEMMY: A vibrator usually. An electric toothbrush I've seen a chick use once – not the bristle side.

TOBY RAND: Beads…. Yeah, anal beads. It's always good. You dip them in baby oil and you insert them in whatever orifice they want and they stay in there for a while and you just fuck around with the rest of their body or whatever and then you just pull them out – slowly, but surely.

VAZQUEZ: It's a tie: I find that the best thing to use on girls usually is a butt plug. It's like a small dildo to put up their ass while you're fucking them from behind. They go fucking bananas with that shit. And what's good about that is that it kind of warms them up for anal if they've never done anal before. Then they start to get used to it and they're like, 'Oh it's not so bad. All those women's magazines are wrong. I actually like this.' Then next thing you know, you're pounding the back door with no problems. So if you use one of those small dildos up their ass while you're fucking them at the same time, they go bananas! The other toy that's a tie with that is the anal beads. What's good about those is that once you put them in, you can fuck them in any position and those things are in there. While that's up their ass, they're getting stimulated and it changes how their pussy feels while you're fucking them, which is great. Usually if I use the beads, I'll fuck her every which way and then I'll fuck her from behind and have her tell me when she's going to come. Then when she's like, 'I'm going to come,' I'll just pull the beads out slowly and dude, it's like fucking fireworks! The Asians figured it out man; they know everything.

Fruit and vegetables – what works best?

ACEY SLADE: Taking them out of the wheelchair.

ADDE: I don't have much experience in that actually, but one time I stuck a strawberry up in my girlfriend's pussy just for fun and we were just laughing about it. It was nothing sexual, but I just stuck it up there and drew it out and chewed on it. It had nothing to do with sex – it was like, 'Let's misbehave!'

ALLISON ROBERTSON: I don't know, I've never tried. I do think that if you're going to have sex, I think fruit is actually good to eat before because it's not spicy or weird and you're not going to have weird breath. I think fruit is really good for your breath, so I think it's sexy to eat fruit before. It's pretty generic – strawberries and shit – but it works.

ANDREW W.K.: I have never engaged with those but that's a really interesting idea. I remember thinking in sex ed class, as it's often portrayed in movies and again in pop culture but also in real life, when they would present bananas and/or cucumbers for people to practise unrolling condoms onto. I thought that was really intense and kind of intimidating, because cucumbers are usually pretty big and a lot of those fruits and vegetables can be pretty intimidating in their size. I can imagine it would be very thrilling with very phallic objects and maybe women use them on their own or we fantasise about women using them on their own, but I've never done it. I've heard of people using other objects like bottles and baseball bats, but I've never gone that route myself.

BLASKO: As far as food goes, I've had some luck with the red vines – a little casual whipping with the red vines. That seems to work well.

BRENT MUSCAT: I guess I'm vanilla. I don't think food is sexy but I guess the whole strawberries and whipped cream could be fun. I've heard of people eating sushi off girls' bodies but for me, I'd rather go and eat good sushi and bring the girl home and have good sex. I don't think they necessarily have to be mixed. Or if you want dessert, eat a nice dessert and go home.

BRUCE KULICK: I've played a little bit with food before, like a little honey, a little strawberries, or this or that. Generally, I haven't done a lot of edibles with my sexual encounters.

CHIP Z'NUFF: I've never tried those. I've talked to people who have tried a few things. The cucumber is a little bit too big. The celery stick I prefer to eat myself to give me a rig, as opposed to putting it inside the woman. There are all kinds of different little tricks. I'm kind of old-fashioned so I'm really not a fruit guy.

DANKO JONES: Nah, I'm not into that stuff. Nothing; it does nothing for me.

DOUG ROBB: I have no idea; I've never used any fruits or vegetables. I'm assuming it'd have to be cucumber-esque and not pineapple-esque.

GINGER: Blindfolded, a woman can be sent to a very wonderful place using juicy fruits to feel and taste.

HANDSOME DICK MANITOBA: Food and sex goes good. I don't do food on a regular basis, but I think that light whipped cream in a can is good because that's fun. You shake it up and spray it – it's sweet and it's light. Food is fun on girls' bodies. I think your brain overloads on pleasure because you're sexually stimulated and then there's sugar, which is like a positive stimulation for your body, so you've mixed a bunch of stimulations. That's a lot of fun sometimes; that's about as weird as I get.

JAMES KOTTAK: I've seen a lot of banana-eating contests in bars, if that has anything to do with it. There's something going on there.

JESSE HUGHES: Giant black cucumbers.

JIMMY ASHHURST: It depends on your partner; you wouldn't want to come out with a pumpkin. Ha! Maybe you would.

LEMMY: I've never done anything with that.

NICKE BORG: Small oranges... that's a recent one I can think of.

ROB PATTERSON: Neither. They're too flexible. (Laughs.)

TOBY RAND: Love the fruit. Being Australian, we love our mangos and if the girl is into mangos, there's nothing better than peeling the skin off a mango, smearing it all over their body and actually using the pip of a mango as a dildo. While you're doing it you can eat it while you're eating her... it's fucking amazing. Whether it be peaches or apricots, just smear yourselves in a fruit that you both enjoy and eat it.

VAZQUEZ: I love food. I've never mixed it into the whole sex thing, like food and sex. But I'm sure it would be amazing – like having some nice roasted pork while I'm going to town on some girl.

Are there any tools or devices that greatly assist in getting aroused?

ROB PATTERSON: Many... many.

TOBY RAND: Yeah, just vibrators mate. I don't know what their names are, but there's a really cool one that's like a bullet. There's nothing cooler than seeing a chick just getting off on a vibrator and just looking you in the eye – just deadly serious.

VIRGINITY

"NOTHING WILL MAKE THE OTHER PERSON WANT TO PERFORM SEXUAL MIRACLES MORE THAN ON A FIRST TIMER"

What is the best way to put a virgin at ease that first time?

ACEY SLADE: I prefer maturity over virginity.

ADDE: Be nice. Go slow, be nice. Be a gentleman.

ALLISON ROBERTSON: I think being sure that they're ready, and gentleness is always good. Also being prepared that they're going to change their mind, because I know girls are always like, 'I'm ready! No I'm not! I'm ready! Get your hands off me!' I think no matter how old you are, the guy has to be ready to be like, 'That's OK. There's no rush.' That's really hard on a guy's end, but that's the tips I would say.

ANDREW W.K.: Well the only time I ever did it was the first time that I had sex. We fortunately both had that to offer one another. That's the best thing you could ever use to put the person at ease, that this is my first time too. If you're going to use that when it's not true, then you're really playing with dangerous elements and building up some very strange karma, but I imagine that's probably the best line: if she's going to lose it then you're going to lose it too. Now, you could also use the line, 'This will be the first time since I lost my virginity.' That nearly is convincing or vulnerable, but it is a first and you could even use that up until the second time, but then you're really starting to grasp at straws. Other than that, it's all going to come down to making her feel loved, and again, if any of it is untrue, you're really playing with dark forces.

BLASKO: Oh man, 'This is going to hurt you more than it's going to hurt me.' Ha! I don't know. That's the reality right? It goes back to being honest; I'm just going to be honest. 'This isn't going to be a party.' I don't know that you can put them at ease.

BRENT MUSCAT: One of my first girlfriends, when we did it, I think she was a virgin. She was so nervous she cramped up and almost went into like convulsions, where her muscles contracted and her hands curled up like claws I remember. I felt so bad. I had to like massage her hands to get them unstuck. She was so frightened and nervous. So I guess if you're a guy and you're with your girlfriend and it's her first time, I think just go slow. A lot of foreplay and just take your time; take it a step at a time. That's the best way I think. If you love them, you want them to feel comfortable.

BRUCE KULICK: Usually those things only happen when you're younger. I might have even done that and I don't remember it; it's been so long. I imagine it probably happened once or twice with me. There's always that concern that a virgin's going to bleed a lot, and nowadays who knows if that is really true because they say, 'Oh, you're breaking the hymen,' but there are girls who use tampons, maybe that's doing it. I don't even know any more. I think that basically any time somebody's going to sexually mature, because that's a big step, being loving and gentle is the best thing. I remember when I was young and I dated someone who was even a little younger than me who wasn't maybe as sexually active. If we turned onto each other… usually the dance is just going to happen and if it's done lovingly, it's all good.

CHIP Z'NUFF: My recommendation is don't go after her. If you find out she's a virgin, leave her alone, because she's going to look at sex as that's the way it's supposed to be all the time. She'll never get over the fact that you're someone who's unselfish and gives her the treatment. I think she'll be looking for a guy like you for the rest of her life. I'm not the guy to take anyone's virginity away and I would talk her out of it. Believe it or not, I really would, because I'm not going to be the one who scars her like that.

COURTNEY TAYLOR-TAYLOR: Be a virgin yourself.

DANKO JONES: For me, honestly, if I'm with someone and I find out she's a virgin, I'll just go, 'Well this date is over. Come back in a couple of years. See you later!' I have no time to be a teacher. It's just annoying and I just don't have fun. Find someone who's also a virgin, lose your virginities together and have some fun experimenting. Get to know your body and be comfortable with your body, then maybe come back and we'll talk. I have no fucking time for that shit! I'm sorry. I don't want to be the one who takes her virginity either. I'm not one of those dudes who collect virginities like people collect baseball cards. I have no time for it.

DOUG ROBB: Just don't pressure her. I think at that point if you're going to be de-virginising someone, whether you are too or not, you basically have to put the ball in their court and let them go at their own speed. If they're ready, they'll do it, and if they're not, you should not be trying to convince them they are. They'll know when they're ready.

HANDSOME DICK MANITOBA: I've never had a virgin, I don't know.

JAMES KOTTAK: I'm from the band Scorpions and we have an album called *Virgin Killer*, so I don't know.

JESSE HUGHES: I recommend Rufenol or Xanax.

JIMMY ASHHURST: Try and convince her that you're one too. Ha!

LEMMY: Fuck her. It's like, 'How do you get a nun pregnant?' Fuck her, right?

NICKE BORG: I did actually have sex with a few virgins and they did come back to me years and years later like, 'Hey, how have you been man? You know what, I'm so glad it was you.' And I'm like, 'Seriously? Are you fucking serious?' 'Yeah, and now I have sex so often.' So the best way I think is the old trick of bullshit. Bullshit her that you do give a shit and they're so young so they go for it. That's fucking horrible and I hate myself for saying this and I will fucking burn in Hell.

ROB PATTERSON: I've never slept with a virgin.

TOBY RAND: The best way is to just talk to her. I think the most important thing I've learned with my sexual partners is to make them feel equal and make them feel like it's fun and there's no pressure. So that adds up to easiness.

VAZQUEZ: A lot of talking, man. A lot of fucking promises! It's been a long time since I've had a virgin and I'm still friends with her to this day. When it comes to anal virginity with girls, I think it comes down to the whole comfort thing. They've got to feel safe with you and that's what virginity is really all about.

Is it better for a virgin to fess up before or after sex?

ACEY SLADE: Definitely before.

ADDE: Please tell me before. That would be better.

ALLISON ROBERTSON: Before I think.

BLASKO: I would probably say before. It really just depends on the individual. Some people are into that and some people aren't, so it depends on the individual situation.

BRENT MUSCAT: I guess it's her prerogative what she wants to do. I think when I was a virgin, I didn't tell the girl I was a virgin. For me, being a guy, I couldn't wait to lose my virginity. I think I was about 15 when that happened and I don't think I told her. I think it's kind of personal and they can say what they want to say.

CHIP Z'NUFF: Well, before probably because you're going to know afterwards when she's in pain. I'm not experienced with virgins, but I've been with them before when they wanted to be with me and I didn't do it because I respected them. I didn't want to be the first guy in the line.

GINGER: Before – absolutely. Nothing will make the other person want to perform sexual miracles more than on a first timer.

HANDSOME DICK MANITOBA: I guess in a way it could be a great turn-on. There's something unique and special about it. Like, I'm thinking back through my life. If I was 21 and somebody said they were a virgin… I think I'd be better equipped to deal with it now as more of a grown-up. I'd be like, 'Relax, take it easy.' If I was doing it now, I'd probably just try to relax her as much as possible, but I think I'd also feel weird or uncomfortable because if she's like 28 it'd be like, 'What's wrong with this woman?' I can't see it happening!

JAMES KOTTAK: I couldn't tell you. I have a 19-year-old daughter, so I can't answer that.

JESSE HUGHES: After, if she's under 18, and before if she's over 18.

JIMMY ASHHURST: By all means before, please. Thank you.

LEMMY: I think they should tell you because depending on your depths of feelings for the girl… I don't think you should deflower somebody you don't feel deeply for.

ROB PATTERSON: Yes!

TOBY RAND: After, I reckon, because then you don't feel quite that bad.

VAZQUEZ: I would say fess up before. Hypothetically, if I was lucky enough to get that… Let's put it this way: fess up if you're 20, but if you fess up when you're like 35, I'm going to run out the door because that would mean that girl is like some religious nut and I'm never going to hear the end of it.

What's the ideal age for someone to lose their virginity?

ACEY SLADE: That's tough because I think kids are growing up so much faster these days. Not only that, but the older I get too… I remember at like 27, having sex with a girl that was questionably 18, and now at 34 I look at 18-year-olds and I'm like, 'God, they're babies.'

ADDE: Tough question. I lost my virginity when I was 14 and I wasn't mature and I wasn't old enough I think, so 15, maybe 16?

ALLISON ROBERTSON: I'd say late high school to after high school is better. I'm a fan of waiting.

ANDREW W.K.: It seems like, from what I've gathered, between the ages of 15 and 16 has been very common. That's what happened for me. They say kids are getting older younger, so maybe it's moved down from that age, but I think that's an age where you've been able to have some time for your sexuality to develop so you can actually have some kind of clue of what to do and how to do it by the time you do it. It just depends on how long you've been sexually active. It varies with each person.

BLASKO: Woah, I don't know man. I'm sure that plenty of my friends that are dads of daughters are going to have a very different opinion of that one... I just want to be realistic and think that when I was young we all lost our virginity when we were teenagers, so I'd have to think not much has changed to now.

BRENT MUSCAT: I think each person's different; each person matures at a different age. A lot of girls these days are losing it at like 13 and I think that's just too young. I just think it's crazy. I'm sure there are girls who lose it earlier than that, but I think ideally if you can wait until you're an adult – 18 would be nice. At least be mature enough that you can handle it. Be mature enough to get on the pill and have condoms and know about sex and you're mature enough to do it. If you're under 18, preferably you'll have someone around the same age and not some old guy.

BRUCE KULICK: I'm older and I think people have pushed the age down and down. Obviously these days, I think being 15 or 16 is no big deal to lose your virginity, whereas when I grew up it was more like 18. I bet you can ask some people who are like, 'No, it's 13 now!' So who knows? I don't have a teenager and if I did I'd be petrified about it. My girlfriend's younger and when we talk about stuff like that, she's coming from a different generation than me, so the information I get is kind of like, 'Huh?' But I kind of knew that too, because you're out there and you know a 16-year-old can be very promiscuous. A) That's fascinating, but B) that's illegal! You don't even want to entertain it, because you realise you can get thrown in jail or have a nice predator record on file because… 'I thought she was 18!' In other words, there are land mines out there for all of us. We're all sexual beings and have sexual desires, needs and wants and that's why a good relationship is a good way to keep you on a healthy path.

CHIP Z'NUFF: I would say 17. This generation is different. There are girls out there way below the age of 17 that are sucking and fucking right now; it's terrible. This new generation is very open-minded and they immediately want to experiment. A guy from my generation would think that it's 17 when guys are starting to learn about it a little, learn about females, but it takes years and years to really learn.

COURTNEY TAYLOR-TAYLOR: I guess kids just have sex earlier and earlier. That's what everyone's been saying as long as they've been saying it, I suppose. I just think 17 or 18 is a really good, respectable age to lose it.

DANKO JONES: From what I've been hearing on the news it's pretty young man. Kids are sending naked photos of themselves and they're underage. There's one case that I know of in America where I think a girl sent naked photos of herself and she got charged with child pornography. I think it's going to get thrown out but that's ridiculous! So I don't know with the age now. I think with kids, 16 or 17 is becoming the average.

DOUG ROBB: Oh man, that's hard for me to say. If somebody had been willing to have sex with me when I was 14, I probably would have, but I didn't until I was almost 18. I don't know; it's hard to say. With sex it's so different for guys than it is for girls and I know there's a large degree of emotional attachment that comes with having sex and being a girl, especially at such a young age. I don't know. I don't think there's a specific age, but it never hurts to wait a little bit.

HANDSOME DICK MANITOBA: Oh, 17, 18. I feel like I'm on a game show – I don't know! It's a guess, because that's the sort of age you're allowed to do everything legally.

JAMES KOTTAK: Well since my daughter is 19, I would say 25.

JESSE HUGHES: The best age to lose your virginity is whatever age you get to leave the house or the street to be selectively alone.

ONE SHOULD DEFINITELY BE AWARE OF LOCAL LAWS IN ORDER TO AVOID ANY SITUATIONS.

JIMMY ASHHURST: The internet can be a valuable tool in that respect. There's a website called ageofconsent.com that I think any self-respecting rock star should be aware of if he isn't already. It's quite, quite interesting. There's certain countries where it's like, 'Fucking hell!' But it's different all around the world. One should definitely be aware of local laws in order to avoid any situations.

LEMMY: Ten. I once had a nine-year-old, but she had the body of an eight-year-old. Well, the ideal age is the age of consent unfortunately.

ROB PATTERSON: Nineteen I would say.

TOBY RAND: Probably 15… 16. Unfortunately it's becoming more like 12.

VAZQUEZ: Dude, if I could have lost it when I was eight then I would have. For guys, it's as soon as possible. For women, if they're smart, they'll probably wait, but they're not all smart about that.

How can that first time be made into a good memory?

ACEY SLADE: I would say don't do it with a band guy, for one. That would be a letdown for sure… or maybe not: I had this experience where I was with these two girls backstage. I was hooking up with them and we were having a three-way. We were doing things and I was about to perform with one of them and put it in and it's not happening. I was like, 'Are you OK?' I thought she had a tampon in or something and she's like, 'Well, we've never done this before.' I thought she meant the three-way thing, so I'm like, 'That's cool, just relax.' So I keep trying and it's still not happening, so I'm like, 'Are you OK?' Then her friend says, 'We're both virgins! We've never done this before!' I'm like, 'Oh my God!' I think that was very memorable for them because I don't think they intended on doing it that night.

ADDE: Long foreplay; a very long foreplay. Maybe the foreplay will go on for weeks… especially for that first one, because just to jump in bed and get drunk and do it is not going to continue anything. So the first time you should really build a long, long foreplay with words and stuff like that. I think I'm a traditional kind of guy.

ALLISON ROBERTSON: I think by having fun and feeling like you're with the right person instead of it being a pressure thing. I think by having fun and hopefully not worrying about parents busting in. To me, sex is more about having fun than seriousness or being scared or pressured. I've always hated that aspect of people pressuring people. That's stupid. It has nothing to do with it.

ANDREW W.K.: Hopefully it's a good memory just from the fact that you did it and it was your first time, but ideally if you're going to be with that person for anything longer than that time that will improve the quality of the context of the memory. I don't know that the first time has to be particularly good or satisfying sexually, but you'd hope that it at least wasn't too painful or traumatic as well. I think doing it in a location that holds some significance will be nice and that you'll have a good vibe with it.

BLASKO: I suppose by just making it as much of a pleasant experience as possible and not being doggish about it, not being a jerk about it.

BRENT MUSCAT: I think for a girl, she should make sure she's dating the guy for a while because most guys just want to have sex. Some guys just want to do it and they'll say anything. 'I love you.' They'll say anything and I know; I've been there and I've done it myself. They'll tell you, 'Oh yeah baby, you're my girlfriend' just to get into their pants. So the most important thing for a girl would be to date the guy for a while and really know about them and take their time to make sure he's not with every other girl. If she can tell him 'No' a bunch of times and the guy's still with her, then the guy obviously likes her, because if he's just there for sex he's not going to wait around.

CHIP Z'NUFF: The first time can be made into a good memory by it not being so X-rated, by spending time with them and talking with them, hanging out and touching and caressing and doing nice things without just running into it immediately and diving into deep water. These kids, once you start fucking, they don't know and you come inside the girl and she gets pregnant and then your whole life changes. So I think the ideal first one would be to hang out, make out a little bit, touch each other, a lot of making out and kissing and it'll lead to more later on.

COURTNEY TAYLOR-TAYLOR: I don't know. My first was not a good memory.

DOUG ROBB: Partially by letting her go at her own pace. Don't buy into the macho aspect of like, 'We're going to fuck and it's going to be wild' and this and that because it's probably not going to be, especially the first time. It takes a while before that type of sex comes around.

JESSE HUGHES: I recommend video tape for making the first time a good memory and it is also very helpful.

JIMMY ASHHURST: Try not to be a fucking asshole. That's a good first step. A key word is always respect, with no matter how you're doing it or whom you're doing it with. Even some of the most degrading acts can be fun if you try and use respect.

LEMMY: It depends on the strength of the hymen. It's going to hurt anyway and sometimes it really, really hurts, so you've got to be sweet with it and careful.

ROB PATTERSON: It can't, it's always awful! Ha.

VAZQUEZ: I guess take your time with them and make them feel comfortable. Make sure the music is right – have a good mix on the iPod.

PREFERRED PARTNER PROFILE

"EVEN SOME OF THE MOST DEGRADING ACTS CAN BE FUN IF YOU TRY AND USE RESPECT"

So there you have it: all the answers from the world's first extensive study of rock stars concerning sex. The sum of their answers paints us a picture of a rock star's typically preferred partner. When their most common answers are profiled, the ideal sexual partner of a rock star presents a woman who:

☐ **Has brunette hair (blonde runs a close second).**

☐ Is endowed with 100% natural breasts, preferably large.

☐ **Is mature (probably aged between 25-35), has no insecurities and oozes confidence.**

☐ Prefers to wear fishnet stockings out, but tight, plain white cotton knickers and a tank-top at home.

☐ **Doesn't have body piercings but maybe a few stylish tattoos.**

☐ Showers daily and maintains her pubic hair with no more than a small landing strip.

☐ **Would be willing to have sex if invited to a band's hotel.**

☐ Understands the importance of condoms.

☐ **Is fine with having her rock star watch her masturbate.**

☐ Loves doggy-style sex and doesn't mind having sex in public sometimes.

☐ **Usually prefers having sex when sober, but is susceptible to a Long Island Iced Tea.**

☐ Owns a Pocket Rocket vibrator for when a rock star's circumcised penis isn't around.

☐ **Would instigate finding another girl for a threesome, if circumstances were right.**

☐ Won't be offended if the rock star doesn't offer his ongoing contact details.

Acknowledgements

All the rock stars that graciously participated in this book and had the guts to candidly spill their beans – thank you!

The team at Omnibus Press, in particular Chris Charlesworth and Norm Lurie for their instant belief and professionalism.

Neil Strauss, Anthony Bozza, Jason Martin, Marta Michaud and the team at Cinematic Management, Kevin 'Chief' Zaruck, Jordan Berliant, Jodi Edmond, Ute Kromrey, Todd Singerman, Shelly Berggren, Pete Galli, Olle Burlin, Kat Sambor, Nicole Gonzales, Adrianne Nigg, Steve Sprite, Sam Norton (for the fateful gift voucher), Peter Landers, and Susan Bridge at the Australian Society of Authors.

And the biggest thanks to my loving wife Sara – forever my darling!

About the Author

Paul Miles is the world's number one historian of one of rock's most reckless and biggest-selling bands: Mötley Crüe. His Chronological Crue website at CrueTime.com, which documents their rock'n'roll lifestyle, has been read well over five million times, and he has self-published five books on the band.

In 2001, he was engaged to analyse the manuscript of Mötley's autobiography for its author. *The Dirt: Confessions Of The World's Most Notorious Rock Band* then spent a record-breaking 10 months on the *New York Times* bestseller list, and he has since performed similar work for its upcoming big-screen Hollywood movie version.

Paul Miles was Executive Producer of the world's first Mötley Crüe tribute CD in 1999, before writing the liner notes for their official *Live: Entertainment or Death* double-album later that year. He's also toured all-access with the Crüe around Australia (2005) and Japan (2008), witnessing life on the road (and in the air).

These experiences, coupled with what he has seen during his seven-hour sets as resident Saturday night rock DJ at Cherry bar in Melbourne's AC/DC Lane since 2005, energised him to make sex and rock come together in a fresh and fun way.

Paul Miles lives in Melbourne, Australia with his wife of 20 years, and the love of his two adult children.

More at www.Paul-Miles.com